Misunderstanding Addiction

Overcoming Myth, Mysticism, and Misdirection in the Addictions Treatment Industry

Micheal M. Pop, MEd

iUniverse, Inc.
New York   Bloomington

Misunderstanding Addiction
Overcoming Myth, Mysticism, and Misdirection
in the Addictions Treatment Industry

iUniverse books may be ordered through booksellers or by contacting:

iUniverse
1663 Liberty Drive
Bloomington, IN 47403
www.iuniverse.com
1-800-Authors (1-800-288-4677)

Because of the dynamic nature of the Internet, any Web addresses or links contained in this book may have changed since publication and may no longer be valid. The views expressed in this work are solely those of the author and do not necessarily reflect the views of the publisher, and the publisher hereby disclaims any responsibility for them.

ISBN: 978-1-4502-0777-5 (sc)
ISBN: 978-1-4502-0778-2 (ebook)
ISBN: 978-1-4502-0779-9 (dj)

Printed in the United States of America

iUniverse rev. date: 7/22/2010

Artwork by Scott M. Pop

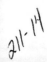

This book is dedicated to my loving wife, Beverly. Over these many years, Beverly has loved, supported, and encouraged me, even when I have given in to my tendency to go against the grain.

Contents

Acknowledgments

There are a number of individuals who have made contributions to my life that, collectively, have provided me with the tools and the opportunities to formulate this book:

Patricia Hurlbut, my mother, who let me loose upon the world and saw to it that I, somehow, made it to adulthood.

Beverly Pop, my wife, who has stood beside me in everything I have tried to accomplish.

Scott Pop, my son, who has always had faith in me.

Elmer Kral, my high school English teacher, who demonstrated that it is acceptable to view the world in a different way.

Yozan Dirk Mosig, PhD, Robert Rycek, PhD, Ken Nikels, PhD, and William Wozniak, PhD, my undergraduate professors, who taught me to think with at least a modest degree of discipline.

William Smith, PhD, and Anna Rodriquez, PhD, my graduate school professors, who allowed me the freedom to make my professional training personally relevant and meaningful.

Allejandro G. Coronado, my former employer and mentor, who taught me to behave like a professional, and who provided me with opportunities to test my thoughts and beliefs in real life.

Ted Gillham, my friend, who has stood beside me through many of life's trials.

Ruben Herrera, JD, my colleague and friend, who has always helped me maintain a sense of humor.

To all these individuals, I offer my undying gratitude.

Introduction

As citizens of the United States, we enjoy the highest standards of living when compared to almost any other collective of people who occupy this planet. The United States boasts the largest and most technologically advanced economy in the world with a median per capita income of $43,800 per year. The average household in the United States has two automobiles parked outside their average $200,000 home. Sixty-six percent of these households have three televisions on which the average American watches more than six hours of programs per day from a selection of more than nine thousand different channels available on cable and/or satellite programming services (U.S. Census Bureau, 2002).

In keeping with those high standards, it is commonly held that people living in the United States pretty much have the best of everything. Among these is access to what many consider to be the most advanced and efficient systems of healthcare in the world. The scientific and technological advancements that have occurred within medicine and other health-care endeavors within just the last one hundred years have increased our life expectancies from forty-seven years in 1904 to nearly seventy-five years, on the average.

Despite the apparent affluence that we in the United States seem to enjoy, there exist many problems that continue to plague us. Among the most obvious is that of the abuse of alcohol and other mood-altering chemicals. One would think that with our apparent affluence, there would be little desire on the part of people living within the United States to want to escape or alter reality. Unfortunately, that does not appear to be the case.

While it seems clear that much of what human beings would need to thrive and to lead happy and productive existences is readily available to individuals within this country, there are many individuals who, for some reason, become trapped in the habitual use of alcohol or other drugs.

The National Council on Alcoholism and Drug Dependence (NCADD, 2005) describes the scope of the problem of substance abuse by citing the following statistics:

- Approximately eighteen million Americans have alcohol problems; about five to six million Americans have drug problems (Institute for Health Policy, Brandeis University, 2001).

- There are more deaths and disabilities each year in the United States from substance abuse than any other cause (Institute for Health Policy, Brandeis University, 1993).

- More than half of all adults have a family history of alcoholism or problem drinking (Brown University Center for Alcohol and Addictions Studies, 2000).

- More than 9 million children live with a parent who is dependent upon alcohol and/or illicit drugs (Ibid.).

NCADD also describes the impact that substance abuse has upon the U.S. economy:

- Alcohol and drug abuse cost the American an estimated $276 billion per year in lost production, health-care expenditures, crime, motor vehicle crashes, and other conditions (Institute for Health Policy, Brandies University, 2001).

- Untreated addiction is more expensive than heart disease, diabetes, and cancer combined (Ibid.). Every American adult pays nearly one thousand dollars per year for the damages of addiction (The White House, 1997).

According to these figures, substance abuse and addictions appear to be among the most pressing concerns that we currently face in our nation. Similar figures resulting from the Substance Abuse and Mental Health Services Administration (Annual Survey, 1998) support these figures.

The Diagnostic and Statistical Manual of Mental Disorders, Fourth Edition, or DSM IV (APA, 1994), describes Alcohol Dependence and Abuse as being among the most prevalent mental disorders within the general population. Estimates offered in that text range from 8 percent of the general population for alcohol dependence to about 5 percent for alcohol abuse in the years 1980 to 1985. In the period 1990–1991, it was estimated that 14 percent of the adult population ranging in ages fifteen to fifty-four years had experienced alcohol dependence within their lifetimes, with 7 percent of that sample having experienced alcohol dependence within the past year.

Looking back just thirty-some years, it was estimated that there were approximately ten million problem drinkers in the United States (Cahalan, 1970). Of that number, the National Institute on Alcohol Abuse and Alcoholism estimated that only five million could be considered to be alcoholics. At about the same time, the National Council on Alcoholism was also claiming that the number of people suffering from alcoholism was somewhere in the vicinity of ten million (Peele, 1989).

Regardless of what estimates are utilized, the appearance is that alcohol and drug problems certainly have not become less prevalent over time. In fact, it appears as if alcohol and drug abuse problems have blossomed at an alarming rate over the last thirty years or so.

What is even more alarming with regard to the ongoing problems of substance abuse and dependence is that these problems have proliferated as they have despite a huge investment that has been made in the development and expansion of services to treat and prevent these problems. For example, the National Center for on Addictions and Substance Abuse at Columbia University (2001) estimated that in 1998, states spent a total of $81.3 billion to deal with substance abuse. Of that amount, ninety-six cents of every dollar spent was devoted to "shoveling up the wreckage of substance abuse" and four cents of every dollar was dedicated to treatment and prevention.

This is an astounding amount of money. Keep in mind that this was only money spent by the states. It does not include private spending or special federal spending. This was only for a period of one year.

If one tries to imagine the amounts of money that have been spent by federal and state governments, coupled with that which has been spent by private citizens in battling substance abuse over the last thirty years, it would amount to an almost unimaginable figure.

So, the question that that comes to mind as we examine our efforts is: why haven't we been able to stem the tide of the ever-increasing alcohol and drug abuse problems in this country? Obviously, there is no easy or singular answer to this ultimate question. It does seem obvious, however, that we have been missing the boat somewhere along the line.

I have been a licensed professional counselor for approximately twenty years. A great deal of my efforts in that period of time, and for some time before I was licensed, had been devoted directly toward working with a variety of populations of people who have suffered from substance use disorders. I have designed and implemented substance abuse prevention programs. I have designed and implemented treatment programs for both adult and juvenile populations. I have also been involved in the development of training programs for beginning substance abuse counselors. In all of these various efforts, I have attempted to devote whatever clinical skills I have to helping people overcome problems that have been directly or indirectly related to substance abuse.

I do not regard myself as the ultimate expert in the field of substance abuse treatment, by any means. Nonetheless, my twenty plus years of providing treatment, intervention, and prevention services in this field have allowed me to garner some insight into the overall problem of substance abuse. As a result of that insight, I have come to believe that we have been mistaken in some of our beliefs regarding why individuals fall prey to mood-altering substances and how substance use disorders can be effectively treated.

In the chapters that follow, I will attempt to outline some of what I perceive to be the most grievous errors that we, as a nation, have made regarding our conceptualization of substance use disorders. I will also offer discussion of how we might benefit from approaching our understanding of substance use disorders from a different perspective.

An attempt will also be made to outline how, in many respects, the approaches that have been utilized over the years to attempt to treat individuals who suffer from substance use disorders have rested on rather dubious assumptions. Evidence will be offered that will indicate that the approaches and methodologies that have been typically applied to treating these disorders have been less than satisfactory in terms of overall results. Alternatives to traditional treatments will be offered.

Facilitation of recovery from substance use disorders may well represent our biggest failure in the addictions field. It is within the efforts made by individuals in their recovery from substance use where it becomes most apparent that we have frequently failed to provide them with the tools and support that these individuals need to be successful in their efforts. It is within this experiential stage of the progression where it becomes obvious that the treatments that have been typically offered to individuals have, in general, been poorly targeted and shortsighted at best.

It is my recognition that some of the discussion that will be offered in this text may be taken to be offensive by some professionals in the field. For that, I can only offer my apologies up front. I will state without reservation that I know that the overwhelming majority of professionals who have chosen to work within the addictions field are kind, caring, compassionate individuals who truly do work arduously to help others overcome their substance use problems. I can say that I offer my views only as part of an effort to improve upon the manner in which we deal with substance use disorders, and, hopefully, improve upon the outcomes of our collective efforts.

The ability to accommodate change is one of the ways we have come to define what is characteristic of mentally healthy individuals. In turn, we should strive to build flexibility into our social institutions and social programs so that the needs of the people of our nation can be met in an ever-changing world. If we have the ability to objectively assess our collective efforts as they have been applied to the understanding and treatment of substance use disorders, we must admit it is past the time that some change needs to occur if we ever hope to stem the tide of our nation's substance use problems.

References

Introduction

American Psychiatric Association. (1994). Alcohol use disorders. Prevalence. (p. 202) *Diagnostic and Statistical Manual of Mental Disorders, Fourth Edition.*

Brandeis University. (1993). Substance abuse: The nation's number one health problem. Institute for Health Policy.

Brandeis University. (2001). Substance abuse: The nation's number one health problem. Institute for Health Policy.

Brown University. (2000). Position paper on drug policy, physician leadership on national drug policy (PLNDP). Center for Alcohol and Addictions Studies.

Cahalan, D. (1970). *Problem Drinkers: a National Survey.* San Francisco: Josey-Bass.

National Center on Addiction and Substance Abuse at Columbia University. (2001). Shoveling Up: The Impact of Substance Abuse on State Budgets. Web site: http://www.casacolumbia. org/absolutem/templates/pressrelease.asp.

National Council on Alcoholism and Drug Dependence. (2005). Alcohol and drug dependence are America's number one problem. Web site: http://www.ncad.org/facts/numberoneproblem.html.

Peele, S. (1989). *Diseasing of America: How We Allowed Recovery Zealots and the Treatment Industry to Convince Us We Are Out of Control.* (p. 47). New York, NY: Lexington Books.

Substance Abuse and Mental Health Services Administration. (1998). *Preliminary Results from the 1997 National Household Survey on Drug Abuse.* Web site: http://www.samhsa.gov.

U.S. Census Bureau. (2002). American Community Survey: 2002. Web site: http://www.census.gov/acs/www. Dept. of Commerce. Washington, DC

U.S. Census Bureau. (2002). Income in the United States: 2002. Web site: http://www.census.gov/prod/203pubs/p60-221.pdf. Dept. of Commerce. Washington, DC

The White House. (1997). National Drug Control Strategy.

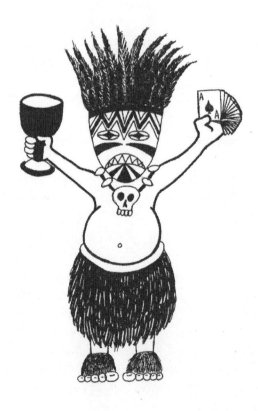

Chapter One

Misinterpretation: The Creation of a Mythical Disease

The prevailing perspective within the addictions-treatment field is that addiction to alcohol and other mood-altering substances is a disease. The definition offered by the National Council on Alcoholism and Drug Dependence (NCADD, 2005) on its Web site states, "Alcoholism is a primary, chronic disease with genetic, psychosocial, and environmental factors influencing its development and manifestations. The disease is often progressive and fatal. It is characterized by continuous or periodic: impaired control over drinking, preoccupation with the drug alcohol, use of alcohol despite adverse consequences, and distortions in thinking, most notably denial."

NCADD further qualifies the definition offered by stating, "Primary refers to the nature of alcoholism as a disease entity in addition to and separate from other pathophysiological states which may be associated with it. Primary suggests that alcoholism, as an addiction, is not a symptom of an underlying disease state."

When one first examines this definition, it seems to provide a rather comprehensive and inclusive way to begin to conceptualize alcoholism. In many respects, it appears to represent plausible understanding of alcoholism as well as addictions to other substances. However, the apparent plausibility of the definition does not necessarily elevate it to be a conceptualization that is factual as opposed to mythical.

There has always been a great deal of contention among professionals in the addictions field as to whether or not alcoholism and addiction to other substances are truly diseases in and of themselves, or if they are a phenomenon that may be more accurately seen as symptoms of some other underlying pathological state. Today, and for probably the last twenty to thirty years, many have actively promoted the notion that addictions represent a diseased state. When asked, most Americans likely refer to addiction as being a disease. In fact, a 1987 Gallup Poll revealed that 90 percent of Americans believe that alcoholism is a disease. So widespread is the notion that addictions are diseases that "people who refuse to accept this concept are often portrayed in the press as being benighted and moralistic" (Peele, 1989).

Well, then, are alcoholism and addictions to other mood-altering substances diseases, or not? Despite the fact that many argue in favor of that notion and that most Americans have come to accept that addictions are diseases, there is much evidence that suggests otherwise. In order to offer an acceptable answer to this question, it might be beneficial to examine some of the evidence that has been utilized to support the disease concept in order to see if such an assumption clearly rests on a solid foundation of scientific evidence.

First, what is a disease? Webster's II New Riverside Dictionary defines a disease as follows: "A condition of an organism that impairs normal physiological functioning."

On a superficial level, it can be clearly stated that the ingestion of alcohol and the introduction of other drugs into the human body does alter the manner in which the body functions. Science has clearly linked prolonged and compulsive use of alcohol to liver damage, heart damage, and malfunctions within the central nervous systems, digestive disorders, and many other physical illnesses. The same can be stated regarding the use of other mood-altering substances as each substance does alter some aspect of human physiological functions. Of course, the same can be said when an individual ingests food. Food does alter the manner in which our body functions. So does the lack thereof.

The same can be said when we take medications that are prescribed by our family physician. The whole objective of taking the medications our doctors prescribe is to alter the manner in which our physical bodies are functioning.

So, does the introduction of some foreign substance into our bodies represent a disease?

If there were to be to agreement that it does, then eating food, taking prescription medications, or simply having a glass of wine with a friend constitutes a disease state. It seems doubtful that we can go so far as to assume that this is what is meant in the definition of disease.

Looking closer at the definition of disease, we must assume that those who propose that addictions represent a disease must be assuming that some "condition" with the human organism must exist that causes individuals to engage in the prolonged and compulsive use of alcohol and/or other substances to the extent that it impairs their physiological functioning. This assumption is, in fact, stated in the definition offered by NCADD. As they have stated, "Alcoholism is a primary, chronic disease with genetic, psychosocial, and environmental factors that influence its development and manifestations."

While this definition in its entirety will be examined at various points throughout this effort, for now, let us just look at portion of that definition. "Alcoholism is a *primary,* chronic disease with *genetic* [emphasis added]" factors that contribute to its development. It is directly stated that alcoholism is a primary disease. That means that the definition itself rests on the assumption that some condition exists within the human body that causes impairment to the normal physiological functioning of an individual. As it is stated, that appears to mean this disease state exists with or without the presence of alcohol. The remainder of that portion of the definition states that it is genetic factors that, in part, cause this condition. In essence, what is being stated is that alcoholism is a disease that is caused, at least in part, by some genetic abnormality or impairment.

Scientific evidence that supported the popular assumptions that a genetic predisposition toward the development of alcoholism might possibly exist began to emerge during the 1970s. The Research Task Force of the National Institute of Mental Health (1975) suggested that alcoholism "runs in families" and that 20 to 30 percent of the children of alcoholics eventually develop alcoholism. This study indicated that children whose parents were alcoholics but who were reared by non-relatives were more likely to develop drinking problems than adopted children whose biological parents were not alcoholics. Other research efforts appeared to support this assumption (Goodwin, 1979 and 1987; Goodwin, et al., 1973 and 1974). It was reasoned that if genetic factors are involved in alcoholism, then the children of alcoholics should show a higher incidence of alcoholism than the children of non-alcoholics (Noble, 1993).

The study of the occurrence of alcoholism among twins also provided impetus for believing that alcoholism was rooted in heredity. An early study comparing concordance rates for alcoholism among identical twins (monozygotic) and fraternal twins (dizygotic) indicated that although identical twins had higher concordance rates, fraternal twins also had high concordance rates (Rosenthal, 1971). Concordance rates are the rate at which a trait expressed in one twin is also expressed in the other. Studies that have examined over sixteen thousand pairs of twins have shown that the concordance rates for alcoholism are higher among monozygotic twins than dizygotic twins (Loehlin, 1972; Hrubec and Ommen, 1981; Pickens et al., 1991).

Family studies have also been utilized to promote the notion that alcoholism is a genetic disease. Rates of alcoholism have been found to be higher in relatives of alcoholics than in relatives of non-alcoholics (Cotton, 1979).

While the results of these research efforts, and that of many other similar efforts, did seem to point to the possibility that heredity may play a major role in the eventual development of alcoholism, they were far from conclusive. When these scientists have discussed the ability to associate heredity as defined within these various studies with the development of alcoholism, the ability to predict how many of these individuals could be expected to exhibit behaviors that are consistent with alcoholism has ranged dramatically. In fact, many of the efforts never offered any predictive estimates at all. On average, such studies as those cited above would suggest that 20 to 30 percent of the children born of a parent who suffered from alcoholism would eventually become alcoholic as well.

The question then becomes what happens to the other 70 to 80 percent of these children?

If alcoholism is a disease that is rooted in some hereditary or genetic abnormality, wouldn't it be reasonable to assume that a much higher percentage of the children being born to alcoholic parents would themselves become alcoholics? While studies such as those that have been referenced do seem to point to a possibility that alcoholism "runs in families," the overall evidence resulting from such studies simply is not sufficient to assume that alcoholism represents a hereditary disease. The best that can be said of the evidence put forth by such research is that when a child comes from a family where one or both parents suffered from alcohol dependence it slightly enhances the possibility that he or she might become alcohol dependent as well.

Perhaps a better question to be asked would be: why is it that 70 to 80 percent of children born to parents that are alcoholics do not become alcoholics?

Over the years, research into the possibility that alcoholism is a genetic disease has become much more sophisticated and intricate. In recent years, scientists have made a claim that they can actually trace the origins of alcoholism to specific genes. In 1990, Blum et al. proposed an association between the dopamine receptor gene (DRD2) and the development of alcoholism. Some studies conducted since that time have failed to demonstrate any association between this specific gene and alcoholism (Johnson, 1996).

Other research has investigated the associations between other genes and alcoholism. Wilhelmsen et al. (2003) studied nine chromosome regions that they believed might be associated with low-level response to alcohol, a factor believed to be involved in the potential development of alcoholism. Their results suggested that chromosomes ten, eleven, and twenty-two appeared to have the strongest relationship to low-level responses to alcohol. While studying the relationship between three receptor genes, Dick et al. (2004) found that only one of three genes studied, GABR3, appeared to have a relationship to alcohol dependence. Urging caution in their findings, the lead investigator of the former study stated, "This suggests that somehow GABA (a major inhibitory neurotransmitter) is involved in these behavioral effects, but we don't know exactly how, so we can't tell what the pathway might be that leads from receptor genes to alcoholism." It was further stated, "A person can carry all kinds of genes that predispose them to alcohol dependence, but if they never take a drink, they won't become an alcoholic."

A person can literally spend years reviewing the volumes of research that has been done in recent years that that has been directed toward finding relationships between genetics and the potential for the development of alcohol dependence and other addictions. Overall, what has been learned from this research is that the exact relationship between our chromosomal makeup and the potential for developing alcoholism is uncertain at best.

After thirty years of increasingly complex research, scientific inquiry has yet to adequately identify the role that genetics might play in alcoholism or addictions to other substances. Yet, proponents of the "alcoholism as a genetic disease concept" rather vehemently will say, "The research all points to a clear association between addictions and genetics." This is clearly an accurate statement. However, an association is not always a good indicator of cause and effect. The leap that is made when an observed association between two phenomena is taken to be a statement of cause and effect is a huge one.

This has been a major problem plaguing the research efforts directed toward making some determination as to what role genetics might have in the development of addictive disorders in individuals. Simply, the overwhelming majority of these efforts have had to rely on basic correlational methodology. Granted, many of the more recent efforts have attempted to employ more advanced statistical methods in efforts to test observations. Nonetheless, at their basis, these have still been simple correlational studies.

For those of you who might not be familiar with research methodology, a correlation is a simple statement that indicates that two variables appear to be related in some way. Frequently, researchers attempt to manipulate, or simply observe, the changes that occur in one variable, which they call an independent variable, and then observe if that manipulation or observed change appears to result in a change in the behavior of the remaining variable, which they call a dependent variable. Any change that occurs is statistically analyzed to determine to what degree there might exist a relationship between variables. That analysis results in what is called a correlation coefficient which is expressed as a coefficient on a scale which is 0 to 1, or a 0 to a -1. A coefficient that equals 1 is said to be a perfectly positive correlation. A coefficient that is -1 is considered to be a perfectly inverse correlation.

It must be remembered that in terms of empirical design, this is a relatively simple process. As such, it is considered to be a non-experimental or what is frequently referred to as a quasi-experimental design. It results only in a statement of a potential relationship or association between two phenomena. Scientists must be very careful not to assume that a cause/effect relationship exists simply because two variables appear to go together. This, generally speaking, is usually just a starting point in the research process.

When researchers observe that relationships appear to exist between two variables, they begin to form more complex and discrete hypotheses. Then, researchers may attempt to devise more stringent ways to test these hypotheses utilizing methods that allow for more control over the variables they are attempting to test and to other variables that might also confound their observations.

Unfortunately, when it comes to testing hypotheses that relate to human physiology and behavior, there are legal, ethical, and moral issues that frequently prevent researchers from being able to go much beyond correlational studies. For example, it is not possible for researchers to manipulate certain biological functions within live human subjects due to the possibility that this might harm the subject. It is easy to imagine that it is nearly impossible to manipulate neurotransmission processes or to manipulate genetic structure directly in living human beings without the risk of causing some harm to the individual.

To illustrate how easy it can be to draw an erroneous conclusion based on the assumption that a correlation might constitute a cause–effect relationship, we can examine some everyday phenomena that may at times appear to be related in some way. Let us compare the sales of snow cones with the occurrence of bicycle accidents for children under the age of fifteen. As we chart these two phenomena, we notice that as the sale of snow cones increases, so does the number of bicycle accidents. If this trend appears to continue to occur over time, we can say that these two phenomena appear to be related. But does one cause the other? Or, does the likelihood that the sale of snow cones increases during the summer months, just at the same time that children under the age of fifteen are out of school and riding their bicycles much more frequently than they do during the winter months, offer a better accounting for the appearance of a relationship between these two distinctly separate phenomena? Even though it may appear that the sale of snow cones has some bearing on the rate at which the bicycle accidents occur, it would seem most likely that there is no real direct relationship between these phenomena.

As one can see, there are many things in life that may appear to have some relationship. That does not mean that any one of these events or occurrences causes a change in something else that we may observe. The same can reasonably be stated when we attempt to assume that alcoholism is caused by some genetic abnormality.

Anyone who has taken a college level biology class learns that the chromosomal makeup of any living organism represents the potentials for growth and development for that organism. For example, two seeds of corn that came from a single ear of corn consist of essentially identical genetic materials. Yet, if we plant these two seeds, will they always grow and develop into identical plants of corn? Not necessarily. It is entirely possible that one seed will grow to be a beautiful corn plant that produces two seemingly perfect ears of corn, while the other, which was planted a few only three feet away from its sibling seed, may grow to be to be a stunted plant that produces nothing. The amount of water, the amount of sun, the amount of fertilizer, and so on, that each of these seeds receives during their respective periods of growth and development will, at least in part, determine how these seeds grow.

Human beings are not that different. We each get a portion of our genetic makeup from our respective parents, who got theirs from their parents, and so on. Simple logic would dictate that if we have siblings, we should look, grow, and act very similar to each other since we each receive our genetic make up from our parents. But, as we all know, it simply doesn't work that way. Even identical twins will frequently have physical features that are sufficiently dissimilar as to make it easy to differentiate between the two. Also, even though they are genetically very similar to each other, it is very likely that they each will possess dissimilar temperaments and personality characteristics. They will likely grow to have interests and ambitions that differ from each other, and so on.

What we do believe we know is that our genetic make up simply holds our potential for growth and development. What we ultimately grow to be as human beings depends on all the many and various events and experiences that can effect our growth and development from the time that we are conceived to the time that we perish.

We are also reasonably certain that no two people that have ever been born are completely identical. We are all generally genetically similar in that we are all human beings. Still, enough genetic variability exists that each of us is in some way unique.

There certainly exists the assumption that no human being ever born on this planet, perhaps save one, has ever been genetically perfect. We are all born with imperfections, and vulnerabilities. As we grow and develop, these imperfections and vulnerabilities become more and more apparent as we live our daily lives. For example, some of us are small in physical stature and lack abundant physical strength while others grow to be large and strong. Some of us have vulnerabilities that can relate to any part of our anatomy, such as our digestive systems, our cardiovascular systems, our muscular systems, and our nervous systems. When we are placed under stress, some of us will react to that stress by experiencing problems with our digestion; we may begin to develop weakness in our cardiovascular systems or our nervous systems, and so on. When we are stressed, we might also become depressed, anxious, or angry in response to whatever we might have experienced.

So, do we assume that these inherent imperfections and vulnerabilities are diseases? Well, in some manner we have to say yes. We all suffer from the inherent disease that we call life. One fact that we all can rely upon is that none of us makes it out of this alive.

It is becoming increasingly apparent that the results of ongoing research efforts intended to determine if alcoholism is a result of genetic abnormality indicate that alcoholism and other addictions could possibly be related to any number of genes that comprise our overall genetic makeup. It may also be that the specific genes that make an individual potentially vulnerable to alcohol and other drugs may vary greatly from one individual to another. This, in effect, was stated by NIAAA Director Enoch Gordis, M.D. (1992). Dr. Gordis stated,

> Progress has been made in understanding genetic vulnerability to alcoholism. We know, for instance, that more than one gene is likely to be responsible for this vulnerability. We must now determine what these genes are and whether they are specific for alcohol or define something more general, such as differences in temperament or personality that increases an individual's vulnerability to alcoholism. We must also determine how genes and the environment interact to influence vulnerability to alcoholism. Based on our current understanding, it is probable that environmental influences will be at least as important, and possibly more important, than genetic influences.

In essence, it seems entirely possible that what we may have assumed to be a disease process rooted in genetic abnormality is likely to turn out to be simply evidence that human beings, each in their own way, do possess imperfections and vulnerabilities.

It is my simple belief that alcoholism and other addictions may each just be one of the ways that these imperfections and vulnerabilities are manifested in individuals. Simply, if alcoholism is a disease that is determined by genetics, then we all suffer from a disease of some similar nature.

Based on the sum total of the evidence that has resulted from the efforts that have been expended over the last thirty years or so to empirically demonstrate that "alcoholism is a primary, chronic disease with genetic factors that contribute to its development," it would have to be stated that there exists very little in the way of empirically derived evidence that offers valid support to such a notion.

Assuming that genetics is a determining factor in the development of alcoholism or other addictions has been, and it still remains, a matter of conjecture. It appears to be more a matter of a myth than it a scientific fact.

Even if we were to find a magic bullet of a gene that predisposes us to alcoholism, what would we do with that knowledge? Would we devise a test to screen infants at birth or before? Would we prevent existing alcoholics and addicts from ever having children? If not, could we possibly shield these children of alcoholics from all the influences that might set them on a path toward alcoholism? Could we manipulate human beings genetically to ensure that they never become addicted to any substances?

If I were to use the analogy that alcoholism and other addictions represent a four-alarm fire, and if we were to attempt to extinguish that fire with a bucket of water that is represented by the assumption that such maladies are the result of a genetic disease or abnormality, I fear that when we go to throw our bucket of water onto the fire, we are not going to even hear much of a sizzle, let alone make much progress in extinguishing the blaze.

Believing that alcoholism or other addictions constitute a primary disease is simply a myth that has been created through the misinterpretation of scientific inquiry.

References

Chapter One

Blum, K., Noble, E. P., Sheridan, P. J., Finley, O., Montgomery, A., Ritchie, T., Ozkaragoz, T. Z., et al. (1991). Association of the A1 allele of the D2 dopamine receptor gene with severe alcoholism. *Alcohol,* **8(5)**, 409–416.

Cotton, N. S. (1979). The familial incidence of alcoholism: A review. *Journal of Studies on Alcohol,* **40(1)**, 89–116.

Dick, D. M., Edenburg, H. J., Howard, J., Xuei, X., Goate, A., Kuperman, S., Schuckit, M., et al. (2004). Association of GABRG3 with alcohol dependence. *Alcoholism: Clinical and Experimental Research,* **28(1)**, 4–9.

Gallup Organization. (1987). Summarized in misconceptions about alcoholism succumb to educational efforts. *The Gallup Report No. 265*, October 1987, 24–31.

Goodwin, D. W. (1979). Alcoholism and heredity. *Archives of General Psychiatry,* **36**, 57–61.

Goodwin, D. W. (1987). Genetic influences in alcoholism. *Advances in Internal Medicine,* **32**, 283–297.

Goodwin, D. W., Schulsinger, F., Hermansen, L., Guze, S. B., and Winokur, G. (1973). Alcohol problems in adoptees raised apart from alcoholic biological parents. *Archives of General Psychiatry,* **28**, 238-243.

Goodwin, D. W., Schulsinger, F., Moller, N., Hermansen, L., Winokur, G., and Guze, S.B. (1974). Drinking problems in adopted and nonadopted sons of alcoholics. *Archives of General Psychiatry,* **31**, 164–169.

Gordis, E. (1992). The genetics of alcoholism—A commentary by the director. *Alcohol Alert.* National Institute on Alcohol Abuse and Alcoholism, No. 18, PH357, July 1992.

Hrubec, Z., and Ommen, G. S. (1981). Evidence of genetic predisposition to alcohol cirrhosis and psychosis: Twin concordances for alcoholism and its biological end points by zygosity among male veterans. *Alcoholism: Clinical and Experimental Research,* **5(2)**, 207–215.

Johnson, K. (1996). The dopamine D2 receptor as a candidate gene for alcoholism. Unpublished thesis. School of Community Medicine University of New South Wales, February 1996.

Loehlin, J. C. (1972). An analysis of alcohol related questionnaire items form national merit twin study. *Annals of the New York Academy of Sciences,* **197**, 117–120.

National Council on Alcoholism and Drug Dependence. (2005). Definition of alcoholism. Web site: http://www.ncadd.org/facts/defalc.html.

Noble, E. P. (1993). The genetic transmission of alcoholism: implications for prevention. *Drug and Alcohol Review,* **12**, 283–290.

Peele, S. (1989). *Diseasing of America: How We Allowed Recovery Zealots and the Treatment Industry to Convince Us We Are Out of Control.* (p. 46). New York, NY: Lexington Books.

Pickens, R. W., Svikis, D. S., McGue, M., Lykken, D. T., Heston, L. L., and Clayton, P. J. (1991). Heterogeneity in the inheritance of alcoholism. *Archives of General Psychiatry,* **48**, 19–28.

Research Task force of the National Institute of Mental Health. (1975). *Research in the Service of Mental Health.* DHEW Publication

No. ADM 75-236. Washington DC: U.S. Government Printing Office.

Rosenthal, D. (1971). *Genetics of Psychopathology.* New York, NY: McGraw-Hill.

Webster's II New Riverside Dictionary. (1984). Boston, MA: A Berkley Book published by Houghton Mifflin, p. 202.

Wilhelmsen, K. C., Schuckit, M., Smith, T. L., Lee, J. V., Segall, S. K., Feiler, H. S., and Kalmijn, J. (2003). The search for genes related to low-level response to alcohol determined by alcohol challenges. *Alcoholism: Clinical and Experimental Research,* **27(7),** 1041–1047.

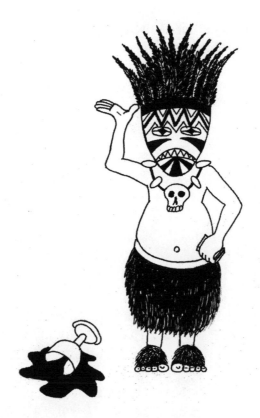

Chapter Two

Misapplication of the Medical Model

Knowing that very little empirical evidence exists to support the notion that alcoholism or other addictions are genetic diseases does not necessarily eradicate the notion that such maladies will still be seen as diseases. People had contended that alcoholism was a disease long before scientists embarked on the investigative journeys that began to relate heredity to alcoholism. Exactly who it was that first articulated the opinion that alcoholism might be most accurately regarded as a disease is not clearly known. Many attribute the first formal articulation of the disease concept to E. M. Jellinek at the Yale University Center of Alcohol Studies. However, evidence of such thought goes back to roughly the same time period that Alcoholics Anonymous was established in the late 1930s.

The book *Alcoholics Anonymous,* commonly called the "Big Book" by those who have become familiar with the organization of Alcoholics Anonymous (AA), was first published in 1939. It is now on its fourth edition (2001). The book outlines the general ideology that forms the basis of AA in addition to the introduction of the Twelve Steps that alcoholics must follow in order to enter recovery from alcoholism. The book also contains the stories of Bill Wilson, a stock broker, and Robert Smith, a physician, who are credited as being the founders of AA. In addition, the book contains the stories of recovery that have been offered by others who have followed the path to recovery that is offered through membership in AA.

The fundamental ideology stated within the Big Book is that alcoholics represent a specific group of individuals who are different from other people in that they are unable, by their very nature, to control their drinking. I, personally, have read through the Big Book many times. There are but a few direct statements to the effect that alcoholism represents a disease contained in that publication. These are contained in the personal stories of those who claim to have found sobriety in AA (pp. 187 and 191). There is, however, frequent reference made to the notion that alcoholics are in some way unique and they can never assume they can live as other people do. In Chapter Three of the Big Book, it is stated that alcoholics are "bodily and mentally different" from others. It is further stated, "We are convinced to a man that alcoholics of our type are in the grips of a progressive illness. Over any considerable period we get worse, never better" (p. 30).

In a sort of preface to the Big Book, a section entitled "The Doctor's Opinion" features a letter written to AA from Dr. William Silkworth, a physician who is believed to have treated Bill Wilson for his alcoholism at the New York City sanitarium. Dr. Silkworth wrote:

> We believe, and also suggested some years ago, that the action of alcohol on these chronic alcoholics is a manifestation of an allergy; that the phenomenon of craving is limited to this class and never occurs in the average temperate drinker. These allergic types can never safely use alcohol in any form at all; and once having formed the habit and found they cannot break it, once having lost their confidence, their reliance upon things human, their problems pile up on them and become astonishingly difficult to solve. (p. xxviii)

While it is not directly stated that alcoholism is a distinct disease in and of itself, it is stated that alcoholics are in some way medically different than other people. For Dr. Silkworth, this difference appeared as some sort of allergic reaction to alcohol that resulted in the alcoholics' experience of constant craving of alcohol for their entire lives. This allergic reaction, according to Dr. Silkworth, is not observed in normal people.

Thus, we have the beginning attempts to create a view of alcoholics as being medically unique individuals, who by their very nature are bodily and mentally different from other people. It is relatively easy to imagine how such a conceptualization could, over time and with slight embellishment, evolve into the definition, such as that which has been promoted by the National Council on Alcoholism and Drug Dependence and other special interest groups.

Unfortunately, it is this view that alcoholics or addicts are somehow bodily and mentally unique, that in my experience has presented one of the biggest obstacles to the treatment of addictions and to the recovery efforts of those individuals who suffer from these afflictions. This will be explained more thoroughly in another section of this literary effort.

Recognition must be given to the fact that prior to the time that Alcoholics Anonymous was established and began to offer assistance to those who suffered from alcoholism, help for such individuals was very hard to come by. Very few organizations were devoted to the provision of any real form of treatment or guidance for alcoholics. There was certainly no scientific consensus as to what alcoholism really was, or how it was most effectively and efficiently treated. Typically, alcoholics would simply present themselves at sanitariums and hospitals suffering from withdrawal symptoms or other medical problems that had been caused by their prolonged drinking. Persons addicted to other drugs had even fewer options for help. Very often, those institutions that did offer assistance to addicted persons were likely to approach the problem as if the addiction was the result of the individual's lack of moral strength or some deficiency of character.

Even those individuals who did secure treatment at a medical facility of some kind received very little in the way of constructive treatment for their addictions. Most often, they received treatment for the medical illness that had been brought on by their compulsive and prolonged use of alcohol or other substances, and then they were released back out into the world with little other guidance aside from being instructed that they should no longer drink or use drugs.

Dr. Silkworth did speak to the lack of understanding of alcoholism that existed prior to the establishment of AA. He said, "We doctors have realized for a long time that some sort of moral psychology was of urgent importance to alcoholics, but its application presented difficulties beyond our conception. What with our ultra-modern standards, our scientific approach to everything, we are perhaps not well equipped to apply the powers of good that lie outside our synthetic knowledge" (p. xxvii). It is made apparent in the remainder of Dr. Silkworth's discourse that he believed AA offered the "sort of moral psychology" which could become beneficial in the treatment of alcoholism.

At this point, I believe that it would only be appropriate to acknowledge the positive contributions that Alcoholics Anonymous has made toward helping individuals in their recovery from alcoholism and other addictions. AA did bring new light to the problem. It also brought what can only be considered as the very first structured approach to helping alcoholics and addicts free themselves of their self-defeating and destructive behaviors. There is little doubt that AA has been helpful to many people in this nation and around the world. It seems likely that AA and other organizations, such as Narcotics Anonymous (NA), will continue to play a role in the treatment of addictions and the recovery of individuals who have suffered from their addictions.

With that said, it must also be stated that AA is just one way to come to an understanding of these problems and to begin to approach the discovery of a possible resolution to the problems of alcoholism and other addictions. It was a starting point. It also has had its limitations. Not the least of which has been its reliance on the concept that alcoholics and addicts are somehow medically and psychologically unique individuals that are doomed to suffer from their illness until the day they die.

Not all alcoholics or addicts have found resolution of their problems in AA or NA. Historically, there has been abundant evidence which pointed out that though many people have been helped by their involvement in AA, an equal or even greater number of people have failed to find resolution to their problems by becoming involved in the fellowship of AA. This should have served as a signal to us that something was missing in this philosophy and app... Unfortunately, we have not moved very much beyond what was conceived nearly seventy years ago. We have been stuck in both our understanding of addictions and the treatment thereof because we have allowed ourselves to fall prey to the notion that alcoholism and other addictions are some form of a disease that is inherent in certain individuals, and whatever form of disease this might be, it is in effect, incurable.

In my opinion, one of the reasons for our failure to move beyond this point has certainly been that as a nation of people, and as professionals in the addictions fields, we have become increasingly dependent on the medical model as a way to understand addictions and as a means to develop treatments for addictions. This is the very model that failed to come to grips with addictions in the first place! Still, we keep hoping upon hope that medical science will provide us with the keys to the Emerald City.

The truth is blatantly evident. Medical science, with its reliance on the reductionistic medical model of understanding of human behavior, has brought us very little with which we can work. This is evident not only with regard to mental disorders in general, but it is specifically evident with regard to alcoholism and other addictions.

As a nation of people, we have come to revere the field of medicine. It is not really a stretch to say that science has become a new religion in our country. We all certainly seem to worship at the altar of science, placing much of our faith in the belief that science, medical science in particular, can make our life longer, healthier, and pain-free. This is perhaps natural for us to do this when you consider all that medical science has been able to offer us within just the last one hundred years. Medical science has been able to eliminate many of the real diseases that, historically, caused humans to die prematurely. Such diseases as polio, small pox, diphtheria, and tuberculosis have been all but eliminated for people living in the United States as a result of medical discoveries. Today, we can expect to live to an age of approximately seventy-five years as opposed to a life expectancy that was just forty-seven years in the year 1904.

...tanding of such illnesses as heart disease has ...oint that treatments and interventions save lives ...now; I'm a beneficiary of such intervention.

...uld deny that medical science has advanced very rapidly ...ast one hundred years. We all in some way benefit from th.. ...ancements. Yet, in some areas that medical science has seen fit to attempt to explore, progress has been very limited. For example, despite the fact that medical scientists have diligently investigated treatments and cures for cancer, it still remains as the number one cause of death for people in this nation. As for alcoholism and other addictions, medical practitioners have little more in their arsenals to fight these disorders than they did seventy years ago.

To exemplify these limitations, let us say that a young man walks into his physician's office and says to his doctor, "I'm worried that I might become an alcoholic." His doctor responds by asking the young man, "Why do you feel that you might become an alcoholic? Do you drink frequently?" The young man responds, "Well, I drink sometimes. But, my dad and my uncles are all alcoholics, and I've heard that alcoholism runs in families. Is there some sort of test you can run to see if I'm in danger of becoming like my dad?"

Obviously, the doctor in the above scenario has but a few options in dealing with this young man. The doctor can take the time and explain his knowledge of alcoholism, which in today's medical environment seems the least likely option, or the doctor will refer the young man to a psychologist or a substance abuse specialist for a drug and alcohol evaluation, which may or may not yield a definitive answer for this young man.

Let's change the scenario to be a little more specific. The young man says, "Doc, I think I'm an alcoholic. I've been drinking a lot lately, and my wife is really upset with me. Is there anything you can do to help me?" Again, we see that the physician is likely to have few options other than to refer the young man to another treatment provider.

Keeping these scenarios in mind, can we still call alcoholism a disease? If it is a disease, it is one that has no established physiological criteria upon which a physician can draw from to make a definitive diagnosis. There are no medical tests that can be initiated to determine whether or not an individual is an alcoholic or a drug addict. There is no medication that a physician can prescribe to reduce this man's symptoms, or to effect a cure. The very best a physician can do is to refer this young man on to another party who will likely attempt to provide the young man with a nonmedical form of treatment.

In 1956, the American Medical Association (AMA) went on record in its recognition that alcoholism is a disease. The problem was then, and it still remains, the AMA has never defined how and why alcoholism, or other addictions, should be considered diseases. Even today, the AMA only offers the following policy statement (H-95-983) entitled "Drug Dependencies as Diseases":

> The AMA 1. endorses the proposition that drug dependencies, including alcoholism, are diseases and that their treatment is a legitimate part of medical practice, and 2. encourages physicians, other health professionals, medical and other health related, and government and other policy makers to become more well informed about drug dependencies, and to base their policies and activities on the recognition that drug dependencies are, in fact, diseases. (AMA, 2005)

Since 1956, the AMA has maintained that alcoholism, along with other drug dependencies, is some form of a disease. Yet, the AMA has never really offered any detailed explanation as to why they consider alcoholism or other drug dependencies to be diseases, nor have they ever claimed to have any cogent method of medically diagnosing, treating, or affecting a cure for these diseases. At the same time, the AMA actively encourages all health professionals, public policy makers, and the government to regard drug dependency as if it is, in fact, a disease. Why should anyone consider drug dependency to be a disease? I know that I have remained mystified by the AMA's directive.

The medical professions have always had a hand in treating alcoholism and other addictions. However, their primary roles have always been to be available to offer treatment to the medical correlates of addiction, such as withdrawal and the organic damage that has resulted from an individual's prolonged use of alcohol or drugs. The medical profession, as a whole, has never been directly involved in the hands-on treatment of alcoholism or other addictions. Yet, physicians or psychiatrists frequently serve as heads of the treatment teams in many of the treatment programs made available to public.

In an attempt to make sense of this, let us examine what exactly medicine has brought to the table in terms of offering direct treatment for alcoholism and other addictions. From 1956, the year that the AMA endorsed alcoholism as a disease, to the present, medical science has produced exactly three discreet treatments for addictions. All three are drugs that have been used in aversion therapies that are sometimes part of a relapse prevention strategy. These three drugs are: tetraethylthiuram disulfide, commonly called Antabuse; Naltrexone; and Acamprosate. That's it, folks! Aversion therapy, sometimes called antagonist therapy, as it has been implemented in the treatment of addictions, consists of the introduction of some medication that either blocks the effect of certain classes of drugs, or it interacts with a substance in such a way as that it causes the individual to experience physical discomfort when a specific substance is ingested by an individual.

Antabuse was actually discovered in the 1930s when workers exposed to tetraethylthiuram disulfide, a chemical used in the rubber industry, became ill after drinking alcoholic beverages. The drug, as it has been used in the treatment of alcoholism, has been prescribed to individuals in an attempt to prevent them from drinking. If a person consumes alcohol within one or two days after taking Antabuse, he or she suffers severe reactions, including nausea, vomiting, and other discomfort. Antabuse has the effect of blocking the progressive breakdown of alcohol so that excessive acetaldehyde accumulates in the body; and acetaldehyde causes dysphoria. Most alcoholics will not consume alcohol after ingesting Antabuse. Those unfortunate individuals who do consume alcohol after ingesting Antabuse risk not only discomfort but in some cases death (Sue et al., 1990).

There has been one primary problem with the use of Antabuse. Simply, it is usually prescribed to individuals for self-administration. Sometimes, the alcoholics just stop taking it.

Naltrexone is a drug that has been used in the treatment of opiate addictions such a heroin. The drug acts to block the normal effects of heroin and other opiate drugs. By blocking the effects of the mood-altering substance, it is believed that because the addict no longer experiences the effect of the opiate to the same degree that they had while actively using the substance, their desire to take the drug will diminish. It has been used with modest success in some treatment efforts. However, Naltrexone has been most often prescribed for self-administration, and its overall effectiveness as a treatment tool is similar to that of Antabuse for alcoholism due to the fact that many of those who are prescribed the drug will sometimes simply discontinue its use (Tai and Blaine, 1997).

Naltrexone has also been used in the treatment of alcoholism, but its overall effectiveness for this purpose has not yet become evident.

The drug Acamprosate has been used in Europe to reduce relapse in weaned alcoholics. Recently, Acamprosate has been approved for use in the United States as well. Acamprosate is a drug that acts on the GABA neurotransmitters in the brain in such a way as to limit the effects of alcohol. Studies have indicated that this is a drug that holds some promise in preventing relapse in recovery from alcoholism (Berton, et al., 1998). Naltrexone and Acamprosate have been used in combination as an aid in relapse prevention with some success as well (Kiefer et al., 2004).

As stated, all three of these drugs have been generally used as a way to prevent relapses during recovery. None of these drugs are used in the initial or primary treatments for addictions. They all suffer from the same drawbacks in that the alcoholics or addicts can simply discontinue using the prescribed drugs and then return to using their drug of choice.

It occurs to me that I did neglect one other form of treatment that was devised and implemented by the medical sciences, that being Methadone treatment for heroin addiction. When thinking about treatment of addictions, I have frequently neglected to remember Methadone maintenance programs, mostly because I have always regarded this approach as being more than just a little nonsensical.

Methadone, a synthetically derived narcotic drug, is prescribed to heroin addicts to decrease the intensity of withdrawal from heroin. Methadone does not produce a euphoric state as does heroin. It was originally believed that Methadone would make it easier for heroin addicts to discontinue their use of heroin. Methadone was thought to be an easy and ready answer to the problem of heroin addiction. Except, the approach has one major drawback: Methadone itself is addictive.

So, there you have the sum total of the direct contribution to the treatment of addictions that medical science has produced since the medical disciplines began to consider addictions to be diseases. Fifty years as a disease and only three drugs. Even then, the primary utility of these three drugs is merely as an aid to prevent relapse, not to directly treat the "disease." And let us not forget Methadone treatment, the treatment approach that simply substitutes one addictive substance for another. This, no matter how you view it, is not a great track record!

Why is it that medical science has failed so miserably in contributing to an understanding of addictions and devising methods to treat what they believe, in fact, to be a "disease"? Part of the problem, I believe, is that medical science relies entirely on the medical model as the primary perspective from which all problems are approached. The medical model is reductionistic in that the primary assumption that forms the foundation of the model is that human beings are no more than the sum of their parts.

This reductionistic thinking and approach is very apparent as we look at exactly how medical science has attempted to understand addictions, and all other abnormal behavior. The primary line of logic is that our genetics determine how our brain functions, and in turn, how our brain functions determines how we behave:

Human beings = Genetics = Brain functions = Behavior.

Simply, we are just the sum of our parts. Just like a machine, only our parts are made of organic materials. According to the medical model, when human beings behave abnormally, it must be happening because of some malfunction of one of our parts.

This line of thinking was very adequately summarized by Ivan Diamond, professor and vice chairman of the Department of Neurology at the University of California at San Francisco. Dr. Diamond stated, "All behavior, thinking, and feeling are controlled by the actions of molecules in the brain. Genes control the proteins which regulate the molecules that carry out all of the functions in the brain. If we could identify genes that confer risk for alcoholism or allow alcoholism to develop, then we could begin to understand which molecules are behaving abnormally, or which molecules are responsible for contributing to alcoholism" (2003).

When this discussion is first examined, it appears to make perfect sense. But, there is a big fly in the ointment that holds this line of thinking together. The very act of introducing alcohol into the human body alters the chemistry within the brain! This is why we become intoxicated! Alcohol doesn't affect just one specific system of neurotransmission controlled by specific genes, it affects them all! Furthermore, the act of adding alcohol, or any other substance, into the human body constitutes an action taken upon the human body by people themselves. It is self-inflicted. It is not controlled by a person's genetics. One would wish to say, "My genes made me do it!" Let's see how well that argument would hold up in a court of law, after someone has been charged with an alcohol-related offense!

This logical plan that is the foundation of the medical model can be traced through nearly all of the medical research that has been devoted to efforts that attempt to offer an explanation as to why human beings sometimes exhibit unusual or abnormal behavior. Utilizing this logic, any abnormal behavior must be caused by "a condition of an organism that impairs normal physiological functioning." Therefore, by definition, all abnormal behavior can be considered to be a disease. Since abnormal behavior is the result of disease, medical science should be able to find a treatment or a cure. And, most likely, this treatment or cure would require that medical science can formulate a medication that will return the body to "normal physiological functioning."

Since it is my intention to limit this discourse, as much as possible, to how the disease concept has been applied to attempts to understand and treat addictions, there will be no attempt to enter into a detailed discussion regarding the contributions that medical science has made in their attempts to explain the broader spectrum of abnormal behavior, or the lack thereof. I will, nonetheless, offer an example of just one case that effectively illustrates how the assumption that an individual's abnormal behavior was the result of disease nearly destroyed one man.

Relatively early on in my career as a mental health therapist, I was working in a rural mental health clinic located in America's heartland. A man, who we will call Dan, came into the clinic stating that he wanted help for his depression. Dan was a highly educated individual who was approaching middle age, and he had been successful in his career in that he had held positions that required him to assume a great deal of responsibility and accountability.

In my first meeting with Dan, our respective levels of educational attainment were an issue. Dan had achieved a doctoral level of education, and I was a master's level therapist. It was clear that Dan really wanted to be seen by someone who had, at least, a PhD. Unfortunately, I was the only one available at the time. Dan and I agreed that we would spend some time getting to know each other, and if he still believed he needed to see a person with higher credentials than I possessed, I would gladly arrange that for him and he would not be asked to pay for my services.

During that first session, Dan informed me that he suffered from "biological depression" and that he had been taking antidepressant drugs for the last twelve years. At that point, I asked Dan who it was who had diagnosed him as suffering from "biological depression." Dan provided the name of a psychiatrist who practiced in a larger city in another part of the state. I also requested his permission to have his psychiatric records forwarded to the agency where I was employed. Dan granted his permission. Also, Dan informed me that he had been hospitalized three times during the last twelve years as a result of experiencing serious depressive episodes. Dan estimated that each of these hospitalizations were of, at least, two weeks duration. All three hospitalizations had occurred in the same city as that in which the psychiatrist had practiced.

During that initial session I also began to gather what is commonly called a psychosocial history, starting as far back in his childhood as Dan could remember up to the present time.

Dan was not suicidal, and he did not appear to be experiencing a level of emotional distress that caused me to become concerned about his overall well-being. So I asked Dan if he would like to make another appointment in a week or two in order to allow me some time to review his records. Apparently, Dan and I hit it off rather well as he agreed to come back for another session in two weeks.

It took about a week for Dan's records to be forwarded to me. As soon as I obtained his records, I set about reviewing his history as it had been documented by his psychiatrist. I noticed that Dan's psychiatrist had been retired from practice for approximately one year.

In reviewing Dan's records, there was documentation as to a treatment plan and documentation as to medications prescribed, periodic medication checks, adjustments to medication, and changes of his prescribed medications. The records also contained documentations of the three hospitalizations. There was no comprehensive assessment or evaluation contained in the record. The initial notation was that the patient had complained of ongoing depression dating back to his early adult years, and that he did not exhibit symptoms of psychosis. It was noted that there was some belief that, initially, Dan had posed a risk for suicide. There was no record of any testing or of any medical examination. The diagnosis offered in the record was simply "Recurrent Depression" on Axis II (?). No additional diagnoses were noted.

The treatment plan, such as it was, simply stated the medications that were to be prescribed to Dan, with the notation that Dan should return for medication checks on a regular basis. There was no recommendation for any other form of therapy. There was no record of any outside referrals for any other therapy.

It was noted that the medications that had been prescribed to Dan changed six times over a period of approximately nine years. That last notation in the record stated that Dan appeared to be stable and that he did not wish to be referred to another physician.

There was little else that was helpful within the record.

After reviewing the record, needless to say, I was more than a little concerned. I asked our agency's psychiatrist to review the record as well, and asked that he inform me as to any conclusions or thoughts that he might have regarding the case.

When Dan returned, we went over his record together. Dan confirmed what had been documented, including the six medication changes. I asked Dan why the medications had been changed. Dan stated, "It seemed like they worked for a while, then after a time, they didn't seem to be working any longer." I also asked about his hospitalizations, about which there was little contained in the record I had received. Dan stated, "I was just there because I was getting real depressed again. They changed my medications, and as soon as they thought I was stable, they let me go."

I then asked Dan two questions that I felt were important. I first asked Dan if he had received any counseling or similar therapy either during his hospitalizations, or at any other time in the last twelve years. Dan replied, "Not in the hospital. I did talk to one guy about four years ago. I didn't think he knew what he was doing so I never went back." I then asked Dan if, during his hospitalizations or in his visits with his psychiatrist, anyone had ever asked him why he was depressed. Dan simply replied, "No."

At that point, I asked Dan if he had any thoughts as to why he had become depressed, initially. Dan sat silent for a few moments. I could sense that Dan wanted to impart something of importance. I could also sense that Dan was really struggling as to whether or not he should say what he was thinking. Ultimately, Dan revealed that he had been sexually molested when he was approximately nine years old. Dan then stated, "I never told anyone about that. My wife doesn't even know about it." I asked Dan if he thought that his depression had anything to do with that experience. Dan stated, "I guess it might. I know that it still bothers me." Dan went on to report that he had experienced recurrent nightmares about that experience, and that when he did allow himself to think about it, these nightmares caused him to feel "very uneasy."

During the remainder of that second session, I gathered the rest of what I believed I needed in terms of his life history. Upon the completion of that effort, I informed Dan of what I believed might have been the cause of his depression and offered him a rough outline of what I thought might be helpful to him. Obviously, since Dan been on medication for twelve years, I also arranged for him to visit with our agency's psychiatrist to discuss his medication needs.

After putting together all the information that was gathered with regard to Dan's case, it became very apparent that Dan had endured a number of rather remarkable and potentially damaging experiences in his childhood years. Dan's family of origin, according to his descriptions, was certainly what would today be considered as being quite dysfunctional.

Dan's father had been physically abusive toward him and his mother. This, in turn, had caused Dan to run away from home at age nine, and he traveled with a carnival troop for approximately three weeks. It was during this time that Dan had been sexually molested, more than one time, by an older male. There were also other experiences that I regarded as being causes for concern.

My diagnosis for Dan was that of posttraumatic stress disorder, with delayed onset, and dysthymic disorder, chronic, with atypical features. The agency psychiatrist agreed with these conclusions. The agency's psychiatrist did recommend continuing medication, which included an antidepressant and an anxiolytic medication. The psychiatrist and I agreed that Dan would need ongoing medication, at least for a time.

I won't go into details regarding the therapy that was provided for Dan. I will simply say that over the course of the next several months, Dan and I worked through many of the issues that I believed were the causes of his emotional distress. The result of that effort was that within a period of four months from his initial visit, Dan was being slowly weaned off his medications. And within eight months, Dan was completely off his medications. Dan continued to do very well without his medications.

My reason for relaying this case history was simply to demonstrate that Dan, for twelve years, had attempted to go through life believing that he had a disease, that being biological depression. The plain truth of the matter was that there had never been any evidence that suggested that Dan had ever suffered from any physiological impairment that would cause his depression. Physically, Dan was in excellent health. And yes, I did insist that Dan complete a thorough medical examination. The result of that examination indicated that Dan was absolutely in good physical health for a man of his age.

Dan was not biologically depressed. Dan did not suffer from a disease. Pure and simple, Dan's emotional discomfort was the result of the experiences that he had endured throughout his life, and the impact that these experiences had on the way that Dan perceived himself and the world around him. Dan simply did not have the skills that he needed to incorporate these experiences, memories, perceptions, thoughts, and feelings into his life in such a way that they did not cause him emotional pain. Once Dan gained these skills, his emotional problems became, at least, manageable without medication.

It is probably true that medication did alleviate Dan's emotional pain for a time. But, ultimately, his reliance on medication only served to prolong his pain. In this instance, a medical professional was attempting to treat a disease that simply did not exist.

The psychiatrist who had previously cared for Dan was a doctor who enjoyed a very good reputation within the state in which we both lived. Because of that reputation, Dan never questioned his doctor's treatment of his problems. Dan had never been given any reason to believe that he might need anything beyond the medication that his doctor had been prescribing to him over the years. Dan did admit, after a month or so of therapy, that he had avoided getting involved in therapy because he did not want anyone to think he was crazy or weak. Dan also admitted that the notion that he had been suffering from a physical disease was much easier for him accept as opposed to the possibility that he might be psychologically impaired in some way. For Dan, that equated to being weak and incompetent.

Unfortunately, Dan's case is simply one of many. Over the course of many years, there have been hundreds of individuals with whom I have had the opportunity to work with in a therapeutic effort that have been told that their emotional problems were caused by some biological defect or malfunction. Of course, in the overwhelming majority of these cases, these biological causes have never been identified in any way. Most of these individuals have been prescribed psychotropic medications by their physicians. The majority of these patients sought therapy only because these medications did not work for them, or if they had alleviated their emotional discomfort for time, they did not prevent their emotional problem from recurring.

Since I recognized that there was some pattern to all of this early on in my career as a therapist, I always made it a point to ask these patients if it was easier for them to accept that they might be suffering from a physical disease and hope that medication might solve their problem, as opposed to accepting that they might be required to face psychotherapy and have to set about finding a way to change some aspect of their life in order to resolve their emotional discomfort. Although the responses that were offered by these individuals varied to some extent, most of them admitted that suffering from a physical disease was easier for them because that meant that that their emotional pain was something that simply happened to them because of a disease, and that it was beyond their control. Essentially, what they were saying is that they did not want to have to change their life in any way in order for the pain to stop. Simply, they weren't responsible for their emotions; they were just sick.

Another problem that I, and many others in both the addictions and mental health fields, have encountered is that there appears to be a persistent tendency for medical practitioners to prescribe psycho-active medications to their patients whenever the patients complain that they are experiencing emotional pain of some sort. Dan's case was certainly an example of how that practice was wholly inadequate, serving only to prolong this man's emotional discomfort. But, many of the drugs that are prescribed by medical practitioners to their patients are also addictive!

There is one example that I ran across this very morning as I was reading the local newspaper. This example consists of a letter written to Dr. Peter Gott, who writes a syndicated column that is distributed to newspapers nationwide:

> Dear Dr. Gott: I am concerned about my 70 year old
> mother who, for many years has taken Xanax as a

sleep aid. She refuses to discuss alternative treatment. What are the long term effects of this medicine?

Dr. Gott's response to this letter included information to the effect that, while Xanax is a mild tranquilizer most often used to treat anxiety, it can be addictive. Dr. Gott goes on to provide his reader with some practical guidance as to how this person's mother might be helped (2005).

The point exemplified is that Xanax is an addictive substance that can be obtained only by a physician's prescription. Clearly, the mother in this instance had become dependent on her medication. One can only wonder why a physician would continue to prescribe this medication "for many years" instead of directing his patient to find another way to resolve her anxiety. Now, the poor woman is not only anxious, she is addicted as well.

Over the years, I have worked with many such individuals who have become addicted to medications that have been prescribed by their physicians. Patients that I have worked with have become addicted to a wide variety of prescribed medications ranging from such highly addictive and potentially dangerous drugs as Oxycotin, Codeine, and other narcotics, to less dangerous drugs, such as Xanax. I am certain that others working in addictions have experienced this phenomenon as well.

As can be seen, overall, medical science has not really made what can be considered as being miraculous contributions to the understanding of what mental disorders, including addictions, are and how they might best be treated. In fact, medical science's persistent tendency to view problems that are clearly not diseases as if they are in fact diseases has sometimes contributed significantly to the problems of some patients.

In the previous chapter, I discussed the research that has been devoted to determining if there is a genetic cause for the disease of addiction. What that review of notable efforts revealed is that there is really no empirical evidence that would support the notion that alcoholism or any other addiction are caused by genetic diseases or defects. It was even noted that some of these scientists are coming to the conclusion that, even if the genes or combinations of genes that might play a role in the development of addictions might someday be reliably identified, environmental factors can be as, or even more, influential in the development of addictive disorders than are a person's genetics.

Scientists have also spent a great deal of effort studying the possible role that specific neurotransmitters play in the development of addictive disorders. As has been the case with genetics, there have been many claims that scientists have identified specific neurotransmitters that they believe might play key roles in the development of addictions. And, just as it has been evident with regard to genetic research, the relationships that might exist between any variety of neurotransmission processes and alcoholism or other addictions remain mostly a matter of speculation. Simply stated, there exists very little in the way of empirically derived evidence that offers valid support to the notion that abnormalities associated with the neurotransmission processes in our brain cause addiction.

I have chosen to forgo an extensive discussion regarding the neurotransmitter research for several reasons. First, the results of these efforts, overall, offer very little that can be used to explain why alcoholism or other addictions should be considered diseases. Second, the medical model upon which all of this research is based assumes that genetics control how neurotransmitters function within the brain. And third, I wish to spare the reader a long, drawn-out discussion of these efforts, since such efforts have provided no evidence that alcoholism or other addictions are, in fact, diseases.

As was stated earlier in this chapter, we as a nation of people have come to revere medical sciences. If you need proof of this, just look at what percentage of our gross national product comes from the money that is spent on medical care. We have developed this reverence because we have become increasingly dependent on the belief that medical science can save us from our diseases, it can prolong our lives, and it can spare us from our pain. To some of this, medical science has performed beyond belief. And to some of this, medical science has offered little beyond hollow promise. The latter reality is exemplified by the assertion that alcoholism and other addictions are diseases that can be treated medically.

The medical model, with it reductionistic perspective as to how human beings function, fails to make its case on a very obvious level that addictions are diseases. The medical model assumes that abnormal behavior results from an underlying physical condition such as genetic abnormality, damage to the brain, or a malfunction of neural processes. This is an assumption, at least in the case of the addictive disorders, that medical research has yet to provide even a modest amount of proof. This weakness is made even more apparent when we consider how little medical science has been able to contribute to our ability to treat the addictive disorders.

> Can we, in fact, realistically consider alcoholism and other addictions to be diseases according to any established medical criteria? The answer to that question is simply no!

The misapplication of the medical model as a primary means to understand alcoholism and other addictions has merely served to perpetuate the myth that substance dependence is a disease.

Is there any harm that can come from simply believing that alcoholism and addictions are diseases? The answer to that question is undeniably yes. The wholesale adoption of the medical model's assertion that addictions are diseases fosters helplessness in the afflicted person by eliminating patient responsibility in the treatment process. Allowing the alcoholic or the addicted person to believe that his or her problems are the result of a disease promotes their reliance on the notion that they can only be effectively treated with appropriate medications or other medical interventions. As has already been demonstrated, medical science offers these individuals almost nothing in the way of treatment. For alcoholics or addicts who already suffer from feelings of helplessness and loss of control, a reliance on the belief that their problems are the result of disease only serves to perpetuate these thoughts and feelings.

Has the belief that addictions are diseases created obstacles to the effective and efficient treatment of problems? Well, ask any active alcoholic or addict why they have been sent to treatment. For the most part, these individuals will admit to just about anything except that they have a psychological problem related to alcohol or drugs. This is what is called denial in the addictions field. If any one of these individuals does admit that alcohol or drugs is a problem for them, the very first thing you will hear them say is, "I can't help it. I have a disease."

References

Chapter Two

Alcoholics Anonymous (2001). *Alcoholics Anonymous: The Story of How More than One Hundred Men Have Recovered from Alcoholism, Fourth Edition.* Works Publishing Company.

American Medical Association (2005). Policy statement (H-95-983) titled "Drug Dependencies as Diseases." Web site: http://www. ama-assoc.org/ama/pub/category/3342.html. Copyright 1995–2005.

Berton, F., Francesconi, W. G., Madamba, S. G., Zieglgansberger, W., and Siggins, G. R. (1998). Acamprosate enhances N-methyl-D-aparate receptor mediated neurotransmission but inhibits presynatic GABA (B) receptors in nucleus accumbens neurons. The Scripps Research Institute, Department of Neuropharmacology and Alcohol Research Center, La Jolla, CA. *Alcohol: Clinical and Experimental Research,* **22(1),**183–191.

Diamond, I. (2003). Commentary and discussion entitled "Chromosomal regions linked to alcoholism may lead to the identification of specific genes." Department of Neurology at the University of California at San Francisco. Dr. Diamond was discussing the results obtained by Wilhelmsen, K. C., Schuckit, M., Smith, T. L., Lee, J. V., Segall, S. K., Feiler, H. S., and Kalmijn, J. (2003). The search for genes related to low-level response to alcohol determined by alcohol challenges. *Alcoholism: Clinical and Experimental Research,* **27(7),** 1041–1047. Web site: http:/ alcoholism.about.com/cs/genetics/a/blacero30716.html.

Gott, P., (2005). Dr. Peter Gott writes his columns for the Newspaper Enterprises Association. Dr. Gott can be contacted c/o United Media, 200 Madison Avenue, Forth Floor, New York, NY 10016.

Keifer, F., Jahn, H., Tarnaske, T., Helwig, H. Briken, P., Holzbach, R., Kampf, P., et al. (2003). Comparing and combining Naltrexone and Acamprosate in relapse prevention of alcoholism. *Archives of General Psychiatry,* **60**, 92–99.

Sue, D., Sue, D., and Sue, S. (1990). *Understanding Abnormal Behavior.* (p. 270). Boston, MA: Houghton Mifflin Company.

Tai, B., Blaine, J., and the NIDA Treatment Workgroup (1997). Naltrexone: An antagonist therapy for heroin addiction. National Institute on Drug Abuse National Institutes of Health: Summary.

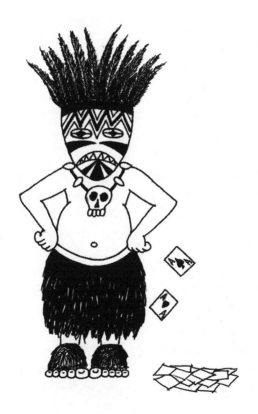

Chapter Three

Misdiagnosis and Miscarriage

In the previous chapters, the evidence that was offered significantly erodes the foundation upon which rests the notion that alcoholism and other addictions are diseases. The truth is that despite all of the efforts that have been made by the medical sciences during the last fifty years or so to convince us that addictions are the result of some disease process, no single or collective group of empirical findings has ever been able to reliably demonstrate a readily identifiable physiological cause for these disorders. There simply is no reason for us to assume that addictions represent distinct "diseases" any more than we would assume that all other expressions of abnormal or eccentric behaviors are the result of disease.

Well, even if addictions aren't diseases as we commonly understand the term disease, what harm is there in saying that an addicted person suffers from a disease? Isn't that just a kinder and gentler way of saying that a person has a problem with alcohol or drugs?

There are many responses that can be given in answer to the two questions asked. In answer to the latter question, yes, this is a kinder and gentler way of making reference to a person who is experiencing problems with alcohol and/or drugs. No one wants to kick a person while he or she is down. No one wants to add stigma to the misery that these individuals might be suffering. On the other hand, even though it might be kinder to assume that a substance-dependent person has a disease, it seems clear that such an assumption would be untrue. In the long run, it seems unlikely that making false assumptions about the source of a person's substance dependence is going to benefit that person in any way.

Answers to the first question are many. First, assuming addictions are the result of disease relieves the individual of any responsibility for his or her problems, in as much as everything that is a source of misery for the individual can, in one way or another, be associated with the "disease." This is a phenomenon that can be observed of any individual who is placed in treatment or who attends AA meetings. If you listen to the dialogues of the substance-abusing individuals, even for just a modest amount of time, it becomes apparent that these individuals associate almost all of the bad experiences that they have ever endured with their "disease."

Second, such assumptions heap a load of helplessness upon the individual. Alcoholics and addicts, in general, all appear to suffer from feelings of helplessness and hopelessness. Believing that their suffering is a result of a disease, these individuals become trapped by something that they believe is totally beyond their control. If they are to ever get help, it must come from a source outside themselves. Since they suffer from a disease, many addicted persons seek some sort of medical or a similar form of treatment. All too often, that treatment is ill-conceived and ineffective.

Third, and most important of all, is that believing that addictions are the result of disease misidentifies the problem. This leads to an inability on the part of treatment providers to devise effective means of helping these individuals. As one of my old psychology professors once said, "If you can't identify what the problem is, how the heck do you ever expect to be able to devise an effective way to treat the patient?"

So that this latter concept is not lost, I will refer back to the case of Dan, which I used to illustrate a point in the previous chapter. Dan suffered ongoing depression for many years. Because Dan's problem was initially diagnosed as originating from some unidentifiable biological source, Dan believed that the only effective treatment for his suffering was that he would have to take antidepressant medication. As far as Dan was concerned, he would likely have to take this medication for the rest of his life in order to avoid yet another devastating lapse into depression. And as was described, this simply didn't work for Dan as evidenced by the fact that Dan continued to experience serious depression despite the fact that he had taken a variety of antidepressant medications over a period of many years. Simply stated, Dan's problem was not accurately identified. Therefore, the treatment devised for Dan did not target the cause of his depression.

Has misidentification of the problem been an obstacle to devising effective treatments for addictions? You can bet the farm that it has! If we take the time to examine how effective the treatments that have been utilized to disrupt the problems of alcoholism and addictions to other substances have been we will see that, by and large, the addictions treatment profession has missed its target in a big way.

Stanton Peele (1989) in his book *Diseasing of America* devoted a great deal of effort to describing how our mistaken beliefs about addictions have created obstacles to our ability to effectively deal with the problem of addictions. Dr. Peele very eloquently stated:

> While I do believe that a host of human habits and compulsions can be understood as addictions, I think the disease version of addiction does at least as much harm as good. An addiction does not mean that God in heaven decided which people are alcoholics and addicts. There is no biological urge to form addictions, one that we will someday find under a microscope and that will finally make sense of all these different cravings and idiocies (such as exercising to the point of injury or having sex with people who are bad for you). No medical treatment will ever be created to excise addictions from people's lives, and support groups that convince people that they are helpless and will forever be incapable of controlling an activity are better examples of self-fulfilling prophecies than of therapy.

It is clear from Dr. Peele's statement that he believes that relying on the disease concept of addictions has certainly not helped our ability to effectively deal with the problem of addiction. In fact, he

40

explicitly stated that the reliance on this concept has done as much harm as good.

With all that said, it is still undeniable that, for some unknown reason, alcoholism and other addictions have always been understood as somehow being different than other mental problems. Historically, alcoholism and other addictions have always appeared to be viewed as being unique problems that confounded medical experts and other professionals who attempted to deal with alcoholics and drug addicts. Dr. Silkworth, in his letter to Alcoholics Anonymous, spoke of being mystified by the problems he encountered as he attempted to treat those who came to his institution for help:

> Faced with this problem, if a doctor is honest with himself, he must sometimes feel his own inadequacy. Although he gives all that is within him, it is often not enough. One feels that something more than human power is needed to produce the essential psychic change. Though the aggregate of recoveries resulting from psychiatric effort is considerable, we physicians must admit we have made little impression on the problem as a whole. Many types do not respond to the ordinary psychological approach. (p. xxix)

Dr. Silkworth is basically stating that his skills as a physician and as a psychiatrist had little impact on the problems of those he had attempted to help. He stated that something beyond human capabilities might be needed in order to help many of the alcoholics that had come to him for help.

In Dr. Silkworth's statement, we see the beginnings of the perception that alcoholism was, indeed, not like any of the other ailments that he had attempted to treat. Alcoholism appeared to be a unique malady that plagued individuals, and it was a malady that seemed resistant to the medical and psychological treatments that were available at that point in time. This perception or, better yet, misperception became much more solidified with the establishment of Alcoholic Anonymous.

Since its inception in 1935, AA has relied on the assumptions that alcoholics were medically and psychologically different from normal people. AA initially referred to this medical difference as being an "allergy" to alcohol that caused an alcoholic to develop an irresistible craving for alcohol. At least one of the personal stories offered in the Big Book refers to alcoholism as being a "terrible disease" (p. 187). According to AA, alcoholics suffer from the "grips of a progressive illness." Additionally, "over any considerable period we get worse, never better" (p. 30). The basic assumption, then, is that alcoholism is a disease and it is progressive and incurable.

Mysteriously, AA's prescription for this disease is generally considered to be more of a spiritual treatment as opposed to a medical treatment. In chapter five of the Big Book it is stated: "Remember that we deal with alcohol—cunning, baffling, powerful! Without help it is too much for us. But there is One who has all the power—that One is God. May you find Him now!" (p. 59).

The Book continues:
Here are the steps we took, which are suggested as a program of recovery:

1. *We admitted that we are powerless over alcohol—that our lives had become unmanageable.*
2. *Came to believe that a power greater than ourselves could restore us to sanity.*
3. *Made a decision to turn our will and our lives over to the care of God as we understood him.*
4. *Made a searching and fearless moral inventory of ourselves.*
5. *Admitted to God, to ourselves, and to another human being the exact nature of our wrongs.*
6. *Were entirely ready to have God remove all these defects of character.*
7. *Humbly asked Him to remove our shortcomings.*
8. *Made a list of all the persons we had harmed, and became willing to make amends to them all.*
9. *Made direct amends to such people wherever possible, except when to do so would injure them or others.*
10. *Continued to take a personal inventory and when we were wrong promptly admitted it.*

11. *Sought through prayer and meditation to improve our conscious contact with God as we understood Him, praying only for knowledge of His will for us and the power to carry that out.*
12. *Having had a spiritual awakening as a result of these steps, we tried to carry to alcoholics, and to practice these principles in all or affairs. (pp. 59 and 60)*

There you have it! This is the prescription that AA has offered to control the terrible, progressive, and incurable disease of alcoholism. A mystical cure for a mythical disease, made more dramatic by the anthropomorphic characterization as the cunning, baffling, and powerful entity—alcohol.

How effective has this prescription been? The plain truth is that there has never, ever been an accurate demonstration as to effectiveness of the twelve-step approach utilized by AA. However, there have been some attempts to offer estimates of how effectively AA has been in its attempt to control alcoholism. What has been revealed by these efforts indicates that AA has a very dismal record of success.

AA's own statistics appear to indicate that its success rate is very low, overall. AA has conducted what it calls Triennial Surveys of its membership since 1977. These surveys measure such membership characteristics as length of membership, age distribution, male–female ratio, employment categories, and length of sobriety. Following their 1989 survey, AA produced a large monograph, "Comments on A.A.'s Triennial Surveys" (AA, 1990) that analyzed the results of all the surveys that had been conducted to that point in time. With respect to the new member drop-out rate, all of the previous surveys were in close agreement. According to the "Comments," the percentages of those coming into AA who drop out after a specified number of months are as follows: 81 percent after one month; 90 percent after three months; and 95 percent after twelve months.

According to AA's own statistics, approximately 95 percent of all persons coming into AA drop out within the first year. Taken at face value, this would provide an estimate that puts AA's maximum success rate at somewhere in the vicinity of 5 percent. This is assuming that all of these persons remained continuously sober during that period of one year.

There have been a number of obstacles that have prevented controlled, scientific investigations into the effectiveness of AA as a treatment for alcoholism. One of these is that AA generally does not open its door to anyone other than its members in order to preserve anonymity. It has also been stated that "AA doesn't like to have researchers around" (Annis, 1987).

One of the more scientifically diligent, and frequently cited, investigations was conducted by Walsh et al. (1991). In this investigation, 227 workers who were identified as being substance abusers were randomly assigned to three different treatment regimens: compulsory-inpatient treatment, compulsory attendance of AA meetings, and the last had a choice of options. The groups were compared in terms of twelve job-performance variables and twelve measures of drinking and drug use during a two-year follow-up period. Their results indicated that there were no significant differences in terms of job performance measures between the three groups. On seven measures of drinking and drug use, the hospitalized group fared the best, and the AA group fared the worst, by comparison. Additional inpatient treatment was required by 63 percent of the AA group, 38 percent of the choice group, and 23 percent of the hospitalized group. The researchers concluded that referral to AA alone or giving their subjects a choice involved more risk than did compulsory-inpatient treatment. The study did not provide any estimate of success rate for any of the three conditions.

In a review of major research efforts that have attempted to determine the relative effectiveness of AA, author Charles Bufe (1998) points out that there are a number of biasing factors that limit researchers' ability to come to exact figures in an effort to determine AA's overall rate of success. These factors might include the definition of what constitutes alcoholism and the characteristics of AA members, such as motivation, socioeconomic class status, marital status, employment, and so on. Bufe states that these factors, and others, may all influence potential outcomes. However, Bufe makes an attempt to provide an estimate of AA's overall success rate by examining the results of many of the more notable research efforts. Bufe provides an estimated success rate for AA that ranges between 2.6 percent and 3.5 percent with the criteria being five years of sobriety. If the criteria for success were lifelong abstinence, as is the stated goal of AA, the success rate would be much lower.

Although it has been very difficult to pinpoint the exact rate of success that can be claimed by AA, it seems reasonably clear that AA's spiritual approach to controlling the terrible, progressive, and incurable disease of alcoholism fails miserably. Actually, it is an outright abomination! It has actually been suggested that at least as many people experience spontaneous recovery from alcoholism as those who have claimed they have successfully followed AA's mystical path to recovery.

Spontaneous recovery, or as it is frequently called spontaneous remission, is a phenomenon that I have observed periodically throughout my career as a therapist. Every once in a while you run across a single patient who, by your best judgment, appears to be very unlikely to ever free himself or herself from addictions. Then, for some reason known only to that individual, he or she stops using the substances that seemed to control every aspect of his or her life. Spontaneously, the individual begins to gradually approximate a more normal pattern of living. I'm sure that most persons who have practiced in the addictions field have observed this apparent spontaneous recovery at one time or another. Sadly, many in the addictions field refuse to acknowledge this as a not-so-rare occurrence.

I do prefer to use the term spontaneous recovery as opposed to spontaneous remission. Remission implies that the individual still suffers from some sort of disease for which the symptoms have merely diminished. And, yes, I do believe that people can recover fully from their addictions. That is, unless they fall prey to the mistaken belief that they suffer from some incurable disease.

Among the very first efforts that provided evidence that spontaneous recovery does, in fact, occur was presented by Charles Winick (1962). Winick observed that most adolescent and young adult heroin addicts outgrew their addictions by the time they reached their mid-thirties. The term Winick coined to describe his observations was "maturing out."

Another study which looked at soldiers who had served in Vietnam and who had become addicted to heroin during their military service yielded results similar to that which is cited above (Robbins et al., 1980). Based on the largest group of untreated heroin addicts ever identified, these researchers observed that many of the addicted soldiers who had been involved in treatment for their addictions upon their returning to the United States did not fare as well in terms of remaining abstinent over specified periods of time as those who did not receive treatment. Robbins and her colleagues stated, "Of those men who were addicted in their first year back, half were treated and half were not.... Of those treated, 47 percent were addicted in the second period; of those who were not treated, 17 percent were addicted." Surprised by their observations, the researchers said, "What we can conclude, however, is that treatment is certainly not always necessary for remission."

An epidemiologist, and strong supporter of AA and of the disease concept of alcoholism, George Vaillant, author of *The Natural History of Alcoholism,* found that among the alcohol abusers he had followed for more than forty years, the majority had overcome their alcohol problem either by cutting back their drinking or quitting altogether. Few of those who had conquered their drinking problems had sought formal treatment. Among those who chose to abstain, more than 60 percent had no contact with AA.

Since observations of spontaneous recovery have been made known within the addictions fields, some researchers have indicated that there appears to be abundant evidence to the effect that alcoholics can outgrow their alcoholism and stop drinking on their own (Tuchfeld, 1981; Stall, 1983). More recently, a large-scale longitudinal study of more than 4,500 adults with prior, significant, and diagnosable alcohol dependence (the National Longitudinal Alcoholism Epidemiology Survey, conducted by the U.S. Census Bureau; Dawson, 1996) reported that twenty years after the onset of alcohol dependence, 90 percent of those who never received treatment were either abstinent or "drinking without abuse or dependence."

One doesn't really have to scour the scientific journals to find evidence that spontaneous recovery to addictions occurs every day. Take addiction to tobacco as an example. I can attest to the fact that breaking the habit of smoking cigarettes is perhaps one of the most difficult of all the addictions to overcome. Most addicts will attest to this as well. Yet, more than forty million people have quit smoking, and according to American Cancer Society, 95 percent of these former smokers have quit on their own.

When one considers that a mere 5 percent (the maximum estimate of efficacy) of the individuals who have attempted recovery from alcoholism by following the "path" which has been prescribed by AA achieve a period of abstinence which approaches five years, combined with the apparent ability that individuals have to spontaneously recover from their addictions, one might begin to wonder why anyone would ever seek formal treatment for their addictions. The truth is most do not! Even if these individuals were to seek formal treatment for their problems, they would, in most instances, just receive an intensified dose of that which is prescribed by AA.

How can we assume that most people who suffer from addictions never seek treatment?

As previously stated, the NCADD estimates that approximately eighteen million Americans have alcohol problems and about five to six million Americans have drug problems. Recent research suggests that only one in ten individuals who need services for alcohol problems actually have received any form of treatment, according to the National Longitudinal Alcoholism Epidemiology Survey, conducted by the U.S. Census Bureau in 1992. Of those who did receive treatment, 33 percent were still abusing alcohol. According to the National Household Survey on Drug Use (SAMSHA, 2000), only 16.6 percent of the persons needing treatment for their drug dependence received that treatment.

As it would appear, only a fraction of individuals who present as being in need of either alcohol or drug treatment ever get the treatment that they need. Fortunately, it does appear that many of these people find some way to either stop using alcohol and/or drugs, or they cut back on their substance use to the extent that it can no longer be considered a problem. It is unfortunate, however, that even for a majority of those who do receive treatment, substance use appears to remain a problem.

Thus far, we have seen that Alcoholics Anonymous as a "path to recovery" is less than effective. At best, 5 percent of all the people who have turned to AA's mystical cure for a mythical disease have found some resolution to their alcohol problems. Apparently, affiliation with AA is about as effective as no treatment at all for most individuals. In fact, it has been observed that individuals who have been offered AA's treatment appear not to do as well as some of those who have never sought treatment for their problems.

Armed with this knowledge, it becomes absolutely befuddling when we come to the realization that almost all of the formal treatment programs that have ever been utilized in attempts to treat alcoholism and other addictions have been based entirely on the twelve-step approach professed by Alcoholics Anonymous and/or Narcotics Anonymous.

The National Treatment Center Study (Roman and Blum, 1997) revealed that 93 percent of drug and alcohol treatment programs in the United States follow the twelve-step approach. The National Survey of Substance Abuse Treatment Services (N-SSATS, 2003; SAMSHA, 2003) indicates that there were 13,623 substance abuse treatment facilities in the United States as of March 31, 2003. The survey also indicated that, at that time, there were 1,092,546 persons receiving treatment for their substance abuse problems.

According to these statistics, of the 13,623 treatment facilities, 12,670 of them base their overall treatment effort on the twelve-step method. And, thus, approximately 1,016,000 persons were involved in twelve-step treatment programs at the time the N-SSATS was conducted.

How effective is the treatment that is being offered by those facilities which rely on the twelve-step method? Offering a definitive answer to this question is, at least, as difficult as describing the overall effectiveness of affiliation with AA. In fact, in many respects, it's more difficult.

One of the most obvious problems that exist with regard to efforts aimed at assessing the effectiveness of twelve-step treatment programs is that most of the programs simply don't attempt to evaluate the outcome of their efforts. For example, according to N-SSATS cited above, only 54 percent of the treatment facilities report that they conduct outcome evaluation of their program by following up with their patients after their discharge. Even then, the majority of these programs are not required to report the results of these outcome evaluations to anyone.

Charles Bufe (1998) pointed out that there have been some difficulties in assessing the overall effectiveness of these treatment efforts:

There have been many studies of twelve-step treatment, but the vast majority are of little use in determining treatment effectiveness for two reasons: 1) they lack control groups; and 2) they were short- or medium-short-term studies. It's impossible to draw meaningful conclusions about treatment's effectiveness without control groups. And any apparent benefits from treatment tend to disappear with time. Thus, long-term studies utilizing control groups are necessary to determining the effectiveness of treatment.

Despite these problems there have been a few efforts that can provide us with some insight. William Miller and Reid Hester (1995) offer the most comprehensive and empirically sound evaluation of treatment methods that can be found anywhere. These authors stated, "We were pleased to see that a number of treatment methods were consistently supported by controlled scientific research." They went on to say, "On the other hand, we were dismayed to realize that virtually none of these treatment methods was in common use within alcohol-treatment programs in the United States." The authors listed approaches that they found to be effective including brief intervention, social skills training, motivational enhancement, community reinforcement approach, and behavior contracting. Twelve-step treatment was not found to be among the effective treatments; but it was noted as being quite likely to be a component of the four modalities that yielded negative results: unspecified "standard" treatment; confrontational counseling; milieu therapy; and general alcoholism counseling. It was also discussed that the authors discovered a significant negative correlation ($r = -.385$) that was found between the strength of efficacy evidence for the modalities and their respective costs; that is, the more expensive the treatment method, the less scientific the evidence documenting its efficacy.

Earlier in this section, reference was made to the National Longitudinal Alcoholism Epidemiology Survey conducted by the U.S. Census Bureau in 1992. One of the other findings that resulted from that effort was that at twenty years after the onset of symptoms of alcohol dependence, 80 percent of those who had undergone treatment were either "abstinent" or "drinking without dependence." But those who had never undergone treatment were doing even better: 90 percent of them were either abstinent or drinking non-problematically. In essence, the results indicated that twice as many of those who had undergone treatment were drinking abusively as those who had never been treated.

The work of George Vaillant (1983) was also mentioned previously. Vaillant followed one hundred patients who had undergone twelve-step treatments over a period of eight years. He then compared this sample to several hundred untreated alcohol abusers. Vaillant discovered that 95 percent of the treated patients relapsed at some time during the eight years that he followed them. Vaillant concluded that "there is compelling evidence that the results of our treatment were no better than the natural history of the disease" (p. 284). Vaillant also added, "Not only had we failed to alter the natural history of alcoholism, but our death rate at three percent per year was appalling" (p. 285).

Perhaps another way in which we can look at the effectiveness of treatment relying on the mystical AA method is to look at recidivism rates. The National Treatment Center Study (Roman and Blum, 1997) which was cited earlier in this section stated that the recidivism rate at the privately owned facilities which were surveyed was 40 percent (p. 17). Common sense would dictate that if these treatment efforts were effective, addicted persons would not need to return to the treatment facility 40 percent of the time.

One could easily assume that the recidivism rate that occurs in publicly funded programs would likely be similar. A report written by a client who had undergone treatment at a VA hospital stated that eleven of twelve patients in his twenty-eight day program had previously undergone inpatient treatment, and that one of these individuals had been in treatment nineteen times (Barton, 1997).

As can be seen, treatment efforts that have been based on the twelve-step method promoted by AA generally have not proven to be any more effective than no treatment at all. As we look back from 1939 to the present day, we see the creation of the mythical notion that alcoholics are somehow unique human beings who suffer from some unidentifiable disease which is incurable. According to popular belief, this is a disease that can only be controlled by adhering to the mystical twelve-step path that is provided through membership in Alcoholics Anonymous or one of its affiliate programs. Despite noble efforts to direct individuals to travel along this mystical path, alcoholism and other addictions have become epidemic because addictions are diseases that are spread within families. This is no one's fault; it's a genetic thing; or maybe it's a brain thing; well, it's most certainly a disease thing. Sadly and tragically, there just aren't enough twelve-step groups and treatment facilities available in an effort to put a stop to the blossoming epidemic. So, in order to stem the tide of this epidemic, it becomes our responsibility as a nation to pool both our public and private resources to create medically directed treatment programs that provide a more expansive dose of this twelve-step treatment. I hope you recognize the fallacious nature of this irrational argument. It is my belief that continuing to do the same thing over and over with the expectation that the repeated behavior will magically bring about a different and desirable outcome is one way of defining insanity.

Now, we arrive at the dawn of the twenty-first century wherein we have more than thirteen thousand private and public treatment facilities in our nation that treat over one million persons for their addictions at any given point in time. Yet, we still face an epidemic of alcohol and drug abuse and dependence. From the statistics that are provided by our nation's prestigious institutions and think tanks, our addiction problems are growing, not receding! Does it occur to anyone that there is something wrong with this picture?

Not only does it appear that clinging to the myth that addictions are diseases has led us to an almost inexcusable misdiagnosis of the problem, it also appears that attempting to cure this mythical disease by taking a stroll down a mystical twelve-step path can only be considered to be a gross miscarriage of a treatment plan!

When one takes the time to look at this sequence of events, one can only shake his or her head and wonder how we got to this point. How is it that we can continue to believe that addictions are diseases when there is, in fact, absolutely no evidence that supports such mistaken notions? How can we continue to believe that the best way to control a malady that is believed to be a disease is by clinging to the mystical twelve-step approach promoted by AA and its proponents?

Considering that there is no reason to believe that our reliance on this approach is any more effective than no treatment at all, how can we continue to pour billions of dollars every year to support treatment programs based on this proven failure-of-a-treatment model?

The only answer that I can reasonably offer is that, perhaps, as a nation we have fallen victim to one of best and most sophisticated misdirection efforts that has ever been devised.

References

Chapter Three

Alcoholics Anonymous. (1939). *The Story of How More than One Hundred Men Have Recovered from Alcoholism.* Works Publishing Company.

Alcoholics Anonymous. (1990). "Comments on A.A.'s Triennial Surveys." No author listed. New York, NY: Alcoholics Anonymous World Services, Inc.

Annis, H. (1987). Is alcoholism treatment effective? *Science,* **236**, 21.

Barton, B. (1997). Twenty-eight days in Wilson's inferno. *Journal of Rational Recovery,* **9(5)**, 17.

Bufe, C. (1998). How effective is AA? *Alcoholics Anonymous: Cult or Cure.* 2nd Edition, revised. San Francisco, CA: See Sharp Press.

Dawson, D. A. (1996). Correlates of past-year status among treated and untreated persons with former alcohol dependence: United States, 1992. *Alcoholism: Clinical and Experimental Research,* **20(4),** 773.

Miller, W., and Hester, R. (1995). What Works? *Handbook of Alcoholism Treatment Approaches: Effective Alternatives.* Boston, MA: Allyn and Bacon.

Peele, S. (1989). *Diseasing of America: How We Allowed Recovery Zealots and the Treatment Industry to Convince Us We Are Out of Control* (p. 4). New York, NY: Lexington Books.

Roman, P. M., and Blum, T. C. (1997). National treatment center study. Athens, GA: Institute of Behavioral Research, University of Georgia.

Stall, R. D. (1983). An examination of spontaneous remission from problem drinking in the Bluegrass region of Kentucky. *Journal of Drug Issues*, **13**, 191–206.

Substance Abuse and Mental Health Services Administration. (2000). National Household Survey on Drug Abuse, 2000. Office of Applied Studies. Web site: http://www.oas.samhsa.gov.

Substance Abuse and Mental Health Services Administration (2003). National Survey of Substance Abuse Treatment Services (N-SSATS) 2003. Web site: http://www. oas.samhsa.gov/2k3/ NSSATS/NSSATS.pdf.

Tuchfeld, B. S. (1981). Spontaneous remission in alcoholics: Empirical observations and theoretical implications. *Journal of Studies on Alcohol*, **42**, 626–641.

Vaillant, G. E. (1983). *The Natural History of Alcoholism*. Cambridge, MA: Harvard University Press.

Walsh, D. C., Hingson, R. W., Merrigan, D. M., Levinson, S. M., Cupples, L. A., Heeren, T., Coffman, G. A., et al. (1991). A randomized trial of treatment options for alcohol abusing workers. *New England Journal of Medicine,* **325(11)**, 777–782.

Winick, C. (1962). Maturing out of narcotic addiction. *Social Problems,* **14**, 1–7.

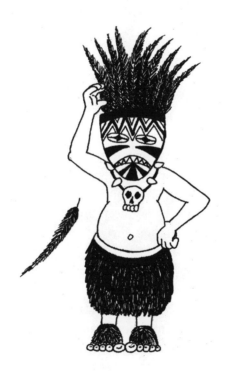

Chapter Four

Misdirection Gets the Key

How is it that the twelve-step "path to recovery" of Alcoholics Anonymous became the standard treatment approach utilized in over 90 percent of the drug and alcohol treatment programs that currently exist? As we have seen from the evidence that was previously reviewed, this certainly did not occur because this mystical approach has ever demonstrated that is has a proven record for successfully treating alcohol- and drug-dependent persons. Nonetheless, Alcoholics Anonymous and its affiliated organizations such as Narcotics Anonymous, through one means or another have been extremely successful in presenting an image that portrays AA as the ultimate authority in terms of understanding and treating all manner of addictions.

Alcoholics Anonymous has grown from being an informal group of just two alcoholics attempting to support each other in recovery in, or around, 1935 to a global organization that boasts a membership into the millions. According to historical data obtained directly from Alcoholics Anonymous, in 1939 there were approximately one hundred sober alcoholics in three founding groups (AA, 2005). The preface to the fourth edition of the Big Book (2001) states that AA had achieved a membership of more than two million persons with 100,800 AA groups meeting in more than one hundred fifty countries around the world (p. xxiii). This, of course, only describes the fellowship of AA. It does not even begin to estimate how AA has influenced the development of the addictions-treatment industry and a host of other organizations that promote AA ideology, conduct research, and otherwise serve to influence how addictions are viewed and dealt with in our nation and in other countries around the world.

As history would make evident, AA's founders, Bill Wilson, and Dr. Robert Smith, were intelligent and capable men who appeared to know how to organize and promote their beliefs and ideas. In addition to the Twelve Steps that were created as a path to recovery, the founders also recognized that in order for their vision to survive, they also had to create an organizational plan to carry their vision into the future and to protect the conceptual identity of their vision. In order for these goals to be accomplished the "Twelve Traditions" of AA were created (pp. 561–566 in the fourth edition), in essence, to devise a formal way to organize AA, to protect the integrity of the organization, and to provide for a public face to promote their ideas and practices.

Later, in 1962, Bill Wilson wrote the "Twelve Concepts for World Services" for the stated purpose "to help ensure that the various elements of A.A.'s service structure remain responsive and responsible to those they serve" (p. 574). These twelve concepts basically provided for the creation of a General Services Board of Trustees to serve as a legal entity to oversee the business interests of AA.

All of this demonstrates a great deal of sophistication for the two individuals who have frequently been portrayed as being hapless and hopeless drunkards who only wanted to do well in helping others. It definitely demonstrates that these men had a vision for the future. And by all accounts, it would seem that their vision has manifested beyond even what they might have imagined.

It is very clear that Bill W. and Dr. Bob, as they are affectionately known within AA's fellowship, knew that they had to gain some legitimate support for their vision. An appendix in the Big Book entitled "The Medical View on A.A." (pp. 569–570) provides evidence that AA had begun to gain to support of the medical community very early on. Comments of support were cited as coming from the annual meeting of the Medical Society of the State of New York in 1944. Statements of support for AA were given by two psychiatrists, Dr. Kirby Collier and Dr. Harry M. Tiebout, and a neurologist, Dr. Foster Kennedy. Also cited as offering endorsement of AA was Dr.

W. W. Bauer, representing the American Medical Association, Chief Psychiatrist of Philadelphia General Hospital, Dr. John Stouffer, and the American Psychiatric Association.

Another appendix, entitled "The Religious View on A.A." (p. 572), states that "clergymen of practically every denomination have given their blessing." There are comments from several prominent clergy showing support from the Catholic and Episcopal churches.

At this point, I will state that I have no real doubts that the intentions of AA's founders were anything but good. There is no reason to suspect that the original mission of AA was to do anything other than provide help to individuals attempting to recover from what they perceived to be a serious and debilitating malady that they called alcoholism. At that point in history, there was truly little else. Attempting to spread their ideas and practices, in my mind, was only a logical next step in their efforts to be of help to alcoholics on a larger scale. What is cited above is provided only for the purposes of illustrating that these men knew exactly how to lay a solid foundation from which they could promote their ideas and practices. It is very clear that AA's founders knew what they were doing in terms of gaining public support and in creating a very favorable public image.

I also must state that just because I acknowledge the original intentions of AA were most likely benevolent, that does not mean that I endorse their beliefs or practices. Like many efforts that have been recorded throughout human history, what frequently starts with good intentions does not always end up that way.

From very early on in its history, AA benefited from the support of both money and power. This is evidenced by the fact that friends of John D. Rockefeller served on the AA's board of trustees which they called the Alcoholic Foundation (AA, 2005). Mr. Rockefeller was known as being a strong supporter of AA. No doubt that such influence contributed to the appearance of articles in *Liberty Magazine* in the fall of 1939, and in the *Saturday Evening Post* in March of 1941. AA claims that their membership roles increased substantially as a result of these favorable articles.

AA has always actively sought support through the various forms of mass media. Although this very much seems to contradict the notion of anonymity which has been perceived as being at the core of AA, this is an organization that has evidenced a remarkable ability to create, for lack of a better term, corporate fronts to promote their methods and philosophy. That AA saw the need to create such fronts in order to distance their spiritual image from real-world business dealings is made evident in their Sixth Tradition (pp. 563–564) where it is stated, "Problems of money, property, and authority may easily divert us from our primary spiritual aim. We think, therefore, that any considerable property of genuine use to A.A. should be separately incorporated and managed, thus dividing the material from the spiritual." That AA intended to promote itself through the media is articulated in their Ninth Tradition as follows: "The trustees of the General Service Board are, in effect, our General Service Committee. They are the custodians of our A.A. Tradition and the receivers of voluntary A.A. contributions by which we maintain our A.A. General Service Office at New York. They are authorized by the groups to handle our over-all public relations and they guarantee the integrity of our principal newspaper, *The Grapevine*" (p. 565).

Very cleverly, AA had been able to create corporate entities to handle its business dealings and public relations activities while preserving its image of being simply a collective of small groups of men and women sitting in smoky rooms concerned only with the issues of sobriety. Charles Bufe (1998) aptly described this as follows:

> But AA's traditions do not forbid, and implicitly encourage AA members to promote AA and its ideology while concealing their AA membership. The eleventh Tradition continues "we need always maintain personal anonymity at the level of press, radio, and films" which certainly seems to encourage both promotion of AA and con-cealment of membership.

Bufe went on to say:

> In fact, such promotion/concealment of identity is very far-reaching. Through it, AA exerts tremendous influence in American society; and AA ideology pervades several important social institutions. Through its members and supporters, AA/twelve-step ideology has great influence in the mass media, legal profession, medical profession, judicial system, penal system, and above all, in the addictions-treatment system.

It seems abundantly clear that since its very inception, AA has had a specific agenda, and it knew how to effectively advance that agenda while protecting its image of benign anonymity.

In 1944, Marty Mann, AA's first female member and a professional publicist, founded the National Council on Alcoholism (NCA) with the assistance of E. M. Jellinek and the Yale Center of Alcohol Studies (Ragels, 1996). The NCA eventually became known as the National Council on Alcoholism and Drug Dependence (NCADD). Since its inception, NCADD has, by and large, acted as the public face of Alcoholics Anonymous, though it claims to have no formal ties to AA. The NCADD has tirelessly promoted the disease concept of alcoholism and the belief that abstinence is the only legitimate treatment goal; it has also attempted to suppress studies on controlled drinking, and has virulently attacked those who publicly disagree with its positions on abstinence and the disease concept (Peele, 1986).

NCADD had actively courted the mass media in the 1950s and 1960s, claiming that it had assisted producers of the Armstrong Circle Theater and the Alfred Hitchcock show in developing early dramatic programs that sympathetically explored the subject of alcoholism. These programs reached vast new audiences in their living rooms and gave NCADD an incredibly influential audience for its message. This, in turn, led to the creation of motion pictures like *The Days of Wine and Roses* (1962), *Clean and Sober* (1988), and *Drunks* (1996) that also portrayed addictions and involvement in AA in a sympathetic manner. It is uncertain as to whether or not NCADD had any advisory involvement in the development of these motion pictures. It does seem apparent that the screenwriters of these film efforts had been influenced by the earlier sympathetic portrayals.

NCADD has also been historically aligned with the medical community. It would appear that AA had the support of the American Medical Association (AMA) and the American Psychiatric Association since its inception. The support of the medical community was made even more solid in 1956 when the AMA went on record and endorsed "the proposition that drug dependencies, including alcoholism, are diseases and that their treatment is a legitimate part of medical practice."

In 1954, the American Society of Addiction Medicine (ASAM) was founded by Dr. Ruth Fox. ASAM, in direct alignment with NCADD, actively campaigned for the disease concept of alcoholism and for abstinence as the only goal for the treatment thereof. ASAM recommended that "physicians and the alcoholism treatment agencies with which they work ... develop relationships of maximum cooperation with self-help groups, such as Alcoholics Anonymous," because "self-help groups, particularly Alcoholics Anonymous, have been a tremendous help in recovery to many thousands of alcoholics, their friends and families" (ASAM, 1979). ASAM has also stated that "expert" physicians should have "knowledge of self-help groups such as AA, NA, Al-Anon, And so on," as well as "knowledge spectrum of this disease and the natural progression if untreated" (ASAM, 1986).

So closely aligned were NCADD and ASAM that the latter actually became a part of NCADD from 1973 to 1984. Even after ASAM separated from NCADD in 1984 the two groups continued to meet annually until 1991, and today they are represented on each other's boards of directors (NCADD, 2005).

NCADD has also aligned with other notable medical organizations that advocate strongly for the disease concept of addictions and involvement in twelve-step programs. NCADD also "offered homes to both the National Nurses Society on Addiction and the Research Society on Alcoholism which, along with ASAM, began publishing the journal entitled *Alcoholism: Clinical and Experimental Research"* (NCADD, 2005).

It is evident that AA's founders had a vision for the future of AA. Through the efforts of members such as Marty Mann, the ideology and practices of AA have been permanently imprinted within American homes and within the very core of America's most influential medical organizations. But, we're not done yet!

In 1970, Senator Harold Hughes, a recovering alcoholic and an alleged AA member, was instrumental in achieving the passage of the Comprehensive Alcohol Abuse and Alcoholism Prevention, Treatment, and Rehabilitation Act of 1970, also known as the Hughes Act. This act established the National Institute on Alcohol Abuse and Alcoholism (NIAAA) and provided for many millions of federal dollars to be devoted to the alcoholism movement. NIAAA then, naturally, contracted with NCADD for guidance and assistance. This, in turn, funneled a great deal of money into the coffers of NCADD.

In 1976, NCADD's budget peaked at about 3.4 million dollars, which was approximately five times what it had been prior to the passage of the Hughes Act (NCADD, 2005). NCADD boasted, "This provided seed money for state voluntary alcoholism associations which in turn helped organize local Affiliates. Marty lived long enough to see how the government had boosted her early vision: the number of Affiliates had risen to an all time high of 223 and their advocacy efforts had helped to bring to at least 23 the number of states who mandated insurance coverage for alcoholism treatment (Ibid.)."

Now we see that the stage was set for the great avalanche of treatment programs that were to be established from the 1970s to the present day. As the federal government began to pour money into the alcoholism movement, NCADD was enabled to push for states to mandate insurance coverage for alcoholism treatment. This ultimately led to insurers such as Blue Cross/Blue Shield, Aetna, Kemper, and others to offer coverage for alcoholism treatment. In response to all the money that was being made available for treatment, the treatment industry came into full bloom.

Prior to the passage of the Hughes Act, the treatment industry was miniscule as compared to what it has become today. Edgar Nace (1993) reported, "From the 1930s through the 1960s, hospitals either overtly rejected alcoholics or subtly deterred them…. The exception was state hospitals. In the 1960s, about 40 percent of admissions to state hospitals were chronic alcoholics.... Private psychiatric hospitals were reporting only 6 percent of their admissions to be alcoholics and very few had specialty units." Nace also noted, "In the place of hospitals, small residential treatment centers, initially located in homes, were formed.... Treatment was informal and followed the principles of Alcoholics Anonymous."

After the passage of the Hughes Act and with influx of money that was made available for treatment by private insurers, the treatment industry expanded very rapidly. The result of the availability of all this federal and insurance money was that by 1982, there were 4,233 alcoholism treatment units; by 1987 the number of treatment units had increased to 5,627; and by 1990, the number had hit 7,766 (Schmidt and Weisner, 1993). As were previously reported, there was 13,623 substance abuse treatment facilities in the United States as of March 31, 2003 (SAMHSA, 2003).

From 1939 to 2003, we can see how effective AA and its promoters such as NCADD have been in to their efforts to shape public opinion through their use of the mass media. Over time, the medical profession, the federal government, and even the medical insurance industry fell into step with the ideology that AA had promoted. In fact, these various entities have all initiated their own efforts to promote the ideas and practices that originated in AA. The overall result of this has been a veritable blossoming of an industry that has been devoted to the treatment of alcoholism and other addictions based solely on the ideology of AA.

There is much more to this history than is evidenced in this effort. My intent is simply to provide some basic insight as to how the ideas and methods that were initially conceived by Alcoholics Anonymous way back in 1939 have formed the basis of nearly all that has been done to address alcoholism and other addictions since.

I must acknowledge that I relied heavily on previous efforts of authors Charles Bufe and Stanton Peele, and a few notable others, in deriving the overall outline of the history presented herein. If the reader is interested in examining a more thorough and extensive recounting of this history, I would encourage the reader to review the works of these authors.

It is undeniable that NCADD has been the most influential of any single entity that has been devoted to promoting the ideas and practices of AA. Sadly though, that is all it has ever attempted to promote. In fact, there is much evidence that suggests that NCADD has actively attempted to suppress views that differ from its own.

> NCADD's stated mission has been to "fight the stigma and the disease of alcoholism and drug addictions."

The organization's efforts are purported to do this by "providing education, information, help, and hope to the public. It advocates prevention, intervention and treatment through offices in New York and Washington, DC, and a nationwide network of Affiliates" (NCADD, 2005). Today, NCADD has more than a hundred affiliate organizations throughout the United States. Typically, these affiliate organizations are referred to as being "councils." Like their parent organization, these local councils exist primarily to carry out NCADD's overall mission of promoting AA, and nothing else.

Earlier in my career in the addictions treatment field, I assisted in the formation of a local council on alcohol and drug addiction, and I also spent some time serving on its board of directors. This council was not affiliated in any way to NCADD. Proudly, I can attest that this council attempted to provide educational, informational, preventive, and early intervention programming that was very diverse in its approach to the issues of addiction. Simply, it did not rely entirely on the philosophy and practices of AA.

I also, for a short period of time, served as an executive director of a local "Council on Alcoholism" that was affiliated with NCADD. This council did rely entirely on AA doctrine in the services it offered to the public. Among the services this agency provided was that it distributed literature, most of which came directly from NCADD, and it offered books and other materials for sale on topics which included alcoholism, drug addiction, treatment, etc. One thing that I can attest to is that absolutely nothing that did not fully endorse AA and its ideology, or twelve-step treatment and recovery, was made available to the public through that council. While serving in the capacity that I did, an overt attempt was made to broaden the scope of services and improve upon the information that was being made available to the public through the agency. I can't say I made much progress with those efforts.

Recognizing that affiliation with NCADD meant that an "Affiliate Council" must fully support the ideology and practices promoted by NCADD. It was implicit that any thought or practice that significantly departed from that promoted by the mother organization was forbidden if the affiliate intended to remain a part of NCADD's network, a privilege for which each affiliate pays, at least, 1 percent of their total annual revenues as a membership fee. Sadly, I must confess that the affiliate that I worked in was funded, in part, by state and federal tax dollars under the heading of "prevention."

NCADD has not only received direct funding from federal tax dollars, but it also receives financial support from all of its affiliate councils in the form of membership fees, some of which is also likely to have come from state and federal tax dollars. While receiving this financial support, it actively promotes AA ideology solely and discourages the promotion of any other practices or perspectives that may actually be more valid and effective in combating the problems of addiction.

On the surface, AA and its front groups like the NCADD, ASAM, and NIAAA appear to be innocent and benevolent organizations that are only attempting to combat alcoholism and other addictions in the best way possible. When one begins to explore the addictions treatment field in earnest, it quickly becomes clear that AA and its promoters have frequently acted as dogmatic tyrants in their attempts to remain in control over the domain that they have dominated for the last seventy years or so.

One perspective that adherents to the AA ideology have vehemently opposed and attempted to suppress is that it is possible to treat alcoholism through what is called a "controlled-drinking approach." Such approaches generally have a primary treatment goal of reducing the alcohol-dependent person's alcohol use to the point wherein it no longer represents a problem to the person's day-to-day functioning. You will remember that the only goal deemed appropriate by AA is that of total abstinence; a goal that, according to much evidence, is rarely achieved.

Mark and Linda Sobell (1973) published two empirically sound papers that demonstrated that bad-prognosis alcohol abusers given moderation training tended to fare better than a similar group given abstinence training. The Sobells were immediately attacked by disease-concept advocates and harassed to the point that they were forced leave the United States and seek employment in Canada.

Mary Pendery, the Sobell's primary persecutor, along with Irving Maltzman and L. J. West, published an article in the 1982 journal of *Science* in an attempt to discredit the findings generated by the Sobell's work. In fact, they literally accused the Sobells of fraud in their research effort. According to Stanton Peele (1986), "An earlier version of the *Science* article (which the journal rejected on the grounds that it was libelous) had been widely disseminated to the media. In several of interviews, at least one of the article's authors repeated his claim that the Sobells had committed fraud." A panel convened by the Addiction Research Foundation which investigated the allegations of fraud on the part of the Sobells cleared them of any wrongdoing.

In 1983, *60 Minutes* aired a report on the Sobell's study which was strongly sympathetic to Pendery et al.'s claim that the Sobell's works were fraudulent and damaging to alcoholics' efforts to overcome their disease. A tape of this program was continuously on display at the NCADD's (then NCA) 1983 convention at which Ms. Pendery delivered an emotionally charged speech criticizing controlled drinking and those who might advocate such an approach to treating alcoholics.

Author Stanton Peele reported that after he defended the Sobell's work in an article he wrote in *Psychology Today* in 1983, his column in the *U.S. Journal of Drug and Alcohol Dependence* was dropped; Mary Pendery attacked him in the speech she gave at the NCA convention in 1983; an invitation to deliver the keynote speech at the Texas Commission on Alcoholism's summer school was withdrawn (and then reinstated after Peele protested); and the number of invitations he had received from conferences like that in Texas dropped dramatically (Peele, 1986). This served as an indication that those who assert views that are in any way in opposition to AA and its fronts can expect severe repercussions.

Peele commented on his experiences by stating:

> Apparently, those in the field had given up expecting freedom of speech or that a range of views should be represented at conferences receiving governmental funding and conducted at major universities. What I uncovered was a matter-of-fact acceptance that those who do not hold the dominant view will not be given a fair hearing; that even mention that there is doubt about accepted wisdom in the field endangers one's ability to function as a professional; and that government agencies reinterpret results of which they disapprove from research they themselves have commissioned. (Ibid.)

Interestingly and sadly, an end to this story of contention between Pendery and anyone who would support the Sobell's efforts came to pass in 1994 when Mary Pendery was murdered by an alcoholic lover. Ms. Pendery left her position as director of the alcoholism treatment program at the VA hospital in San Diego and relocated to work at the VA hospital in Sheridan, Wyoming. Ms. Pendery had been romantically involved with a man named George Sie Rega whom she had first met in San Diego. When Sie Rega joined Pendery in Wyoming he was in serious alcoholic relapse. Sie Rega shot Pendery while in an intoxicated state and then shot himself.

An earlier report on controlled drinking called the Rand Report (Armor, Polich, and Stambul, 1978) was met with a similar hysterical response by the NCA. The Rand Corporation Report, which consisted of findings on outcomes at the National Institute on Alcohol Abuse and Alcoholism treatment centers, initially released its report in 1976.

The authors of that report concluded that those who were in remission at eighteen months were as likely to drink without problems as to maintain stable abstinence. Commenting on NCA's response to this report, Don Cahalan (1987) stated, "After valiant year-long attempts by prominent NCA members to have the report suppressed or drastically revised in its findings, it was finally released by Rand in June 1976." After the report was actually released, the NCA made a concerted attempt to criticize and discredit the report.

Cahalan described NCA's criticism stating, "The NCA's major press conference criticizing the report revealed a level of anxiety and anger much higher than ordinary concern about fairness and balance in scientific reporting. NCA officials charged that many alcoholics would be 'dying in the streets' as a direct result of publication of the report." Of course, history has made evident that the NCA's concerns did not come to pass.

It is apparent that AA and its front groups become extremely defensive and reactive to any perspective that might offer a challenge to that which they promote. Charles Bufe in his book (1998) speaks of what he calls "The Web of Influence":

> AA is far from being the innocent organization that most people believe it to be. The familiar gatherings of coffee-slurping, cigarette-smoking ex-drunks are only the tip of the iceberg. AA and its disease-concept of alcoholism dominate the alcoholism treatment industry in this country. Through its hidden membership and its carefully cultivated benign image, AA has tremendous influence in the media. It has powerful "educational" and "medical" front groups such as NCADD and ASAM, that to a great extent, determine the direction of alcoholism research, treatment, and education. (The NIAAA, for example, has funded no controlled drinking research for a decade.) AA's front groups and hidden members vilify and blackball critics and independent researchers. AA and twelve-step treatment advocates attempt to smother alternative treatment approaches. AA's friends and hidden members in EAPs, diversion programs, the judiciary, and penal system coerce probably half a million Americans per year into AA attendance and/or twelve-step treatment....

> This comprises AA's hidden structure and hidden influence. It is, quite simply, a national disaster.

Amen to that!

I do have some personal experience when it comes to being blackballed because of my refusal to toe the AA line. Soon after I became involved in the treatment and prevention of substance abuse problems, I applied for a position as an addictions counselor in an inpatient treatment program that was part of a relatively large corporation specializing in running psychiatric hospitals. By that time, I had been in the addictions field for approximately three years. I had been a licensed professional counselor for more than two years.

When I had applied for the position, I really had little expectation that I would be called for an interview. It had been my previous experience that my professional qualifications exceeded that of most alcohol and drug treatment program directors. From experience, I knew that most of these individuals were very reluctant to hire someone who had more education than they possessed.

Much to my amazement, I was called for an interview. I arrived at my interview appointment on time and was directed into the office of the treatment program director. The very first question that I was asked was, "Are you in recovery?" I responded by stating that I had experienced problems with alcohol earlier in my life, but I had abstained from alcohol use for more than ten years. I could tell that my response was not what the program director desired to hear due to the frown on his face. The gentlemen then asked, "Do you attend AA?" I responded by stating that I did have some experience with AA. Again, I could see that this was not what the director wanted to hear. The director then went on a very long verbal discourse to the effect that he would never even consider hiring someone who he did not believe was, as he called it, "working their own ongoing program of recovery." When the director completed his exhortation, I simply responded by saying that I felt quite comfortable with my life at that point in time and that I was confident that I could be helpful to individuals attempting to rid themselves of their addictive behaviors. That pretty much concluded the interview.

As you might have guessed, I never heard back from that program. I never even got the usual letter thanking me for my interest and informing me that another person had been selected to fill the position. I assumed my refusal to spout the verbiage which would have signaled that I was a fully indoctrinated, hardcore twelve-stepper had eliminated me from consideration.

Since this program was located in a relatively small community wherein I knew most of the other people who might apply for that same position, I was able to find out who had been hired to fill that position. The individual that had been given the position was far less qualified than I; this individual had far less experience in the addictions field; and the individual had not yet acquired a professional credential of any kind. The individual who was hired for this position was, however, a self-professed "recovering person" who did attend AA meetings on a regular basis.

By the time the program director had asked me his first question, I was able to assume that he held the belief that only "recovering alcoholics" could treat practicing alcoholics. As the interview proceeded, it became clear that to be a "recovering alcoholic," one had to religiously attend AA and adhere to the belief that twelve-step treatment was the only way to treat addicted persons. These were the qualifications that this program director was seeking. After nearly twenty years of working in the counseling and addictions treatment field, I am well aware that there are many treatment program directors that employ similar standards when making personnel decisions for the programs they administer.

I have had other experiences in addition to that above. Actually, I have had many. But, I see little purpose in dragging the reader through all of them. I will share one other personal experience that exemplifies the closed-minded and exclusionary attitude that many individuals whom have been indoctrinated by AA appear to possess.

As previously described, I had worked for a short period of time as the director of an NCADD affiliate council. One of the services provided by the agency was that they sold AA medallions and other official AA items. Frequently, AA members who were charged with leading meetings would come into the agency to buy such items. As such, it didn't take long for me to determine the "who's who" within a local AA community.

One day a gentleman who is considered to be among the elite of the local AA community came into the store looking for a specific item. Elite status, within this community, was generally only conferred upon those individuals who have had many years of sobriety and have continued to attend AA religiously. As for this particular gentleman, I was well aware that he had been attending AA for at least thirty years.

On this given day, I was the only person in the agency. The other employees were either out to lunch or working outside of the office. I recognized this gentleman and introduced myself. The man, in return, politely offered his hand without speaking. The man then stated, "I heard there was a new director here. Are you a friend of Bill's?" In response, I simply stated, "Yes. But, I try to be friendly with everyone." No words can describe the expression that my response brought to this man's face. The gentleman was obviously dismayed. He very quickly paid for the items he came to purchase and exited the agency as fast as he could without uttering another word.

This man continued to come into the agency from time to time thereafter. However, I did notice that he would only come into the agency at times when the agency receptionist was at her station to assist him with whatever he might want or need from the agency. Despite the fact that I made an overt effort to always greet this man in a pleasant manner whenever I saw him in the agency, he never spoke a single word to me again. He would simply nod his head to acknowledge my greeting, and quickly carry out whatever was required to complete his business within the agency. I also noticed that, after that first encounter with this gentleman, I was treated much more cautiously by some of the other regulars.

Throughout my career in the addictions field, it has been very apparent that AA with its disease concept and its mystical twelve-step treatment approach was truly "the only game in town." Anyone who did not openly subscribe to that ideology was either totally excluded, or simply tolerated as being the outsider. Tolerance, however, is only granted to those who do not attempt to rock the boat by offering a challenge to the AA doctrine. This is not only true on a local level.

It is apparent that this is how the game has been played on a national level as well.

As was made evident in the previous chapter, more than 90 percent of all the alcohol and drug treatment programs that exist within the United States are based solely on the ideas and practices that have been promoted by AA and its front groups. We can also see that this reality did not happen simply by chance; it happened by design. AA, through its front groups like NCADD, ASAM, and others, and through its hidden membership, has been able to influence the mass media, the medical community, the insurance industry, the federal government, state and local governments, and the judiciary in such a way that ensured that the majority of the alcohol and drug treatment provided in this nation would rely entirely upon AA ideology. It is equally evident that AA and its promoters want it to remain that way.

So the keys to the Emerald City go to AA and its promoters! AA has become the great and wonderful Wizard of the Emerald City, who by virtue of its infinite wisdom has the only true conceptual understanding of this disease called addiction. By virtue of its compassionate heart and advanced spiritual development, only AA can direct us to the mystical path which must be traveled in order to control this mythical disease. Additionally, as can plainly be seen, AA has demonstrated the virtuous courage to see to it that everyone continues to believe that this is true.

Unfortunately, as was portrayed in Frank Baum's story *The Wizard of OZ*, the great Wizard's only real talent was that of misdirection. He was merely able to trick the inhabitants of the Emerald City into believing that he was a great and wonderful wizard, and that they needed him to lead and protect them. The Wizard put on an impressive show for the people. But, in reality, he was just a "humbug." When it came time to truly help someone, like Dorothy, he had nothing in his bag of tricks that would really be of help to anyone. He tried but ultimately failed. In the end, Dorothy had to rely on her own resources to solve her problems. Even the fellowship provided to her by the Scarecrow, the Tin Man, and Cowardly Lion was of very little solace to Dorothy when it came time for her to truly face her dilemma.

> *Myth*: Addiction is a disease. *Mysticism*: The application of a mystical twelve-step path is the only real way to treat the disease of addiction. *Misdirection*: AA and its promoters' ability to convince a nation that only they have the answers.

This "humbug," in its entirety, must be overcome if there is ever to be any hope of coming to a clear understanding of the problems we call alcoholism and addiction to other drugs. Furthermore, myth, mysticism, and misdirection certainly cannot serve as a foundation for formulating treatments to be implemented in an effort to help individuals overcome substance use disorders.

References

Chapter Four

Alcoholics Anonymous. (2001). *The Story of How More than One Hundred Men Have Recovered from Alcoholism. Fourth Edition.* Alcoholics Anonymous World Services, Inc. New York.

Alcoholics Anonymous (2005). Historical data: The birth of A.A. and its growth in the U.S. and Canada. Website: http://www.alcoholics-anonymous.org.

American Society of Addiction Medicine. (1974). Resolution on self-help groups adopted by ASAM board of directors in October, 1979. Web site: http://www.207.181.5/ppoll.htm#Abstinence.

American Society of Addiction Medicine. (1986). How to identify a physician recognized for expertise in diagnosis and treatment of alcoholism and other drug dependence. Adopted by the ASAM board of directors in February 1986. Web site: http://www.207.181.5/ppoll.htm#Abstinence.

Armor, D. J., Polich, J. M., and Stambul, H. B. (1978). *Alcoholism and Treatment.* New York, NY: Wiley.

Bufe, C. (1998). AA's Impact on Society. *Alcoholics Anonymous: Cult or Cure.* 2nd edition, revised. San Francisco: See Sharp Press.

Cahalan, D. (1987). *Understanding America's Drinking Problem.* (p. 135) San Francisco, CA: Jossey–Bass.

Nace, E.P. (1993). Impatient treatment. Marc Galanter, (ed)., *Recent Developments in Alcoholism,* (Volume 11, p. 430).

National Council on Alcoholism and Drug Dependence. (2005). Information gathered on Web site under the locations entitled History and Affiliates. Web site: http://www.ncadd.org.

Peele, S. (1983). Through a glass darkly: Can some alcoholics learn to drink in moderation? *Psychology Today*, April 1983, 38–42.

Peele, S. (1986). Denial—of reality and of freedom—in addiction research and treatment. *Bulletin of the Society of Psychologists in Addictive Behaviors*, **5(4)**, 149–166.

Ragels, L. A. (1996). Prohibition, alcoholics anonymous, the alcoholism movement, and the alcoholic beverage industry. *Journal of Rational Recovery*, **8(4)**, 23.

Schmidt, L., and Weisner, C. (1993). Developments in alcoholism treatment. Marc Galanter, (Ed.), *Recent Developments in Alcoholism*, (Volume 11, Table 1, p. 371).

Sobell, M., and Sobell, L. (1973). Alcoholics treated by individualized behavior therapy: One year treatment outcomes. *Behavior Research and Therapy*, **11**, 599–618.

Sobell, M., and Sobell, L. (1973). Second year treatment outcomes of alcoholics treated by behavior therapy: Results. *Behavior Research and Therapy*, **14**, 195–215.

Substance Abuse and Mental Health Services Administration. (2003). National Survey of Substance Abuse Treatment Services (N-SSATS) 2003. Web site: http://www. oas.samhsa.gov/2k3/ NSSATS/NSSATS.

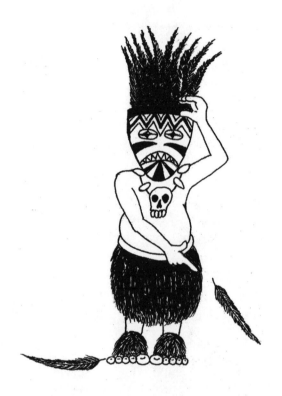

Chapter Five

Misanthropy: Indoctrination, Not Treatment

Despite the fact that the twelve-step approach promoted by AA and its front groups has never proven to be an effective way to treat addictions, it remains that more than 90 percent of the treatment programs that exist today still rely on this utter failure of a treatment model. It is a demonstrable fact that AA doctrine is so predominant within the addiction treatment field that most individuals who practice in the field cannot even imagine that alternatives to the twelve-step method of treatment might actually exist, let alone imagine that some of these alternatives might be more efficacious than the antiquated model which has been put into practice since the late 1930s. As was discussed in the previous chapter, this is a dominance which has been carefully and artfully crafted by those individuals and organizations who have spent their solitary and collective efforts promoting the AA doctrine to ensure that what was to considered to be appropriate treatment for alcoholics and addicts should be based entirely on the concepts and methods that originated in AA.

Before we continue a discussion of treatment, it might be beneficial to define two terms that are frequently used with confusing interchangeability in the addictions fields. The first is "treatment." Treatment, according to *Webster's New Riverside Dictionary*, means the "medical application of remedies so as to affect a cure." The second term is "recovery." According to the same defining source, recovery means "to regain normal health, control, or balance."

When looking to overcome any disease, there is a sequential progression, or order, in which these words should be properly used.

First, there is the onset of a disease. This usually means that an individual begins to exhibit symptoms that signal they suffer from a specific disease. In order to stop or disrupt the progression of a disease, a treatment is applied. Once the treatment has been applied and the disease has been either stopped or cured, then recovery begins and continues, hopefully, until the individual regains normal health. It must be pointed out that if a disease is not curable and can only be arrested, the potential for recovery may be limited by a number of factors. An example of such limiting factors might include the amount of organic damage that was sustained as a result of the disease.

It will be reiterated that the Twelve Steps of Alcoholics Anonymous has been touted as a way to "recover" from the disease that is called alcoholism. Yet, the twelve-step model promoted by AA is the only model utilized in more than 90 percent of all existing treatment programs as the primary means of "treating" this so-called disease! It would seem that with regard to addictions, we can simply skip the treatment part of this sequence and go directly from the onset of the disease to the recovery! Might we be reasonable to assume that this omission on the part of the treatment industry might, at least in part, provide us with some insight as to why we have failed to make much progress in our ongoing battle with substance abuse and substance dependence? Can we even consider that the twelve-step model represents a viable treatment option which has a chance of affecting a cure or of stopping the progression of substance use disorders?

Since it apparent that the twelve-step model is what has been, thus far, considered to be the preferred treatment, let us take a good look at what this prevailing twelve-step model of treatment really does. Let's look at how these Twelve Steps are utilized in the treatment of alcoholism and drug addiction, and then see if we can make some sense as to why this method should be considered to be the preferred treatment method in an effort to stop the progression of these so-called diseases.

It is believed that first application of the Twelve Steps of AA in a treatment effort was likely to have occurred in 1939 when Dr. Robert Smith (co-founder of AA) used the approach he and Bill

Wilson outlined in the Big Book in his work with alcoholics at St. Thomas Hospital in Akron, Ohio (Alcoholics Anonymous, 1989). It was estimated that Dr. Bob treated more than five thousand people at that hospital prior to his death. There is an account describing the treatment that Dr. Bob applied during his efforts in Akron which was offered by a patient called Bill D.: "There was the identification with them [Bill Wilson and Dr. Bob], followed by surrendering his will to God and making a moral inventory; then, he was told about the first drink, the 24-hour program, and the fact that alcoholism was an incurable disease—all the basics of our program that have not changed to this day." It was added that "the alcoholic himself didn't ask for help. He didn't have anything to say about it" (Alcoholics Anonymous, 1980).

As was previously indicated, it does not appear that treatment efforts advanced very much in the period from the 1930s up until the treatment industry began to flourish in the 1970s. As Nace (1993) had reported, "In the place of hospitals, small residential treatment centers, initially located in homes, were formed.... Treatment was informal and followed the principles of Alcoholics Anonymous."

There was one significant development that occurred in 1950s. The Minnesota Model also known as the abstinence model, of addiction treatment was created in a state mental hospital by two young men—one who was to become a psychologist, the other who was to become a psychiatrist, neither of whom had prior experience treating addicts or alcoholics. The model spread first to a small not-for-profit organization called the Hazelden Foundation and then throughout the country. The key element of this approach to addiction treatment was the blending of professional and trained nonprofessional (recovering) staff around the principles of Alcoholics Anonymous (AA). There was an individualized treatment plan with active family involvement in a twenty-eight-day inpatient setting and participation in Alcoholics Anonymous both during and after treatment (Anderson, et al., 1999).

Hazelden and the Minnesota Model have since become synonymous. Hazelden has come to be considered as one of the largest and most prestigious single, private organizations that devotes it efforts to the treatment of addictive disorders. Today, Hazelden offers treatment and continuing-care services, professional education and training programs, international publishing, addiction research, and public policy advocacy (Hazelden, 2004). Hazelden has, throughout its history, also been a very strong promoter of AA. The twelve steps of AA is at the very core of Hazelden's Minnesota Model.

During the 1960s, the Minnesota Model expanded greatly (Hazelden, 1994). After the passage of the Hughes Act in the 1970s, nearly all of the alcohol and drug treatment programs that began to emerge as a result of the money that became available for such treatment were based entirely on this model. In most instances, treatment based on this model had traditionally been provided on an inpatient basis, usually in a hospital-like environment. The typical length of the treatment was twenty-eight days, although there was some variation from one program to another. The cost of this treatment could range anywhere from $500 per day to $1,700 per day (Roman and Blum, 1997). Thus, the total cost of this treatment could range from approximately $14,000 to well over $47,000.

In the late 1980s and on into the 1990s, the insurance industry began to question the costs of this type of treatment when it became clear that the success rates that were obtained from this inpatient treatment were no better than programs offering treatment on an outpatient basis. Insurers and managed-care organizations became increasingly reluctant to authorize payment for the inpatient treatment that had become the standard in the treatment industry. This caused some of these treatment providers to close their programs. However, the majority of the treatment providers that had relied entirely on inpatient programs adapted to these economic changes by offering the same treatment on a less-restrictive and much-less-costly basis such as day treatment or outpatient treatment (Schmidt and Weisner, 1993). Whether the treatment programs were offered on an inpatient or outpatient basis, the treatment programs still relied on the same model of treatment that they had always utilized—the Minnesota Model.

Since there are no dramatic differences in the treatment method employed by the majority of the programs that utilize the Minnesota Model, an attempt will be made to outline the overall goals of this treatment approach, and to describe how these programs purport to achieve these goals. Before we embark upon that task, we do need to look at the issue of detoxification.

Many people believe that that the treatment of addictions consists primarily of detoxification. While this may have been true up to 1939, it is not that way today. Detoxification is frequently achieved in a hospital setting wherein the addicted person is given time to go through whatever withdrawal he or she might experience as a result of his or her discontinuing the use of alcohol and/or other drugs. Typically, this is done under medical supervision and the patient's experience of withdrawal is made more tolerable by the use of a variety of medications (most frequently tranquilizers) administered and monitored by the medical personnel. Detoxification programs may allow the patient anywhere from three to fourteen days to complete the detoxification process, depending on the patient's needs.

Not all patients that enter treatment for their addictions require detoxification. According to SAMHSA (1997), only about 23 percent of those treated for alcoholism in 1995 went through detoxification. From my own experience in the treatment field, very few individuals truly need to go through detoxification programs unless there is evidence that they are indeed physically dependent upon the substance(s) that they have been abusing. Those who have been long-time abusers of alcohol or of narcotics are the most likely to require a period of detoxification.

Detoxification is not a goal of twelve-step treatment. But, there are some treatment programs that routinely require that anyone entering into treatment go through a detoxification program before they are admitted into their treatment programs. One physician, Elizabeth Bartlett, MD (1997), reported her experience of being required to complete a detoxification program prior to her entry into a twelve-step treatment program: "I was placed on 'detox' and medicated, heavily I might add, despite the fact that I had not had a drink in a month and had no physical symptoms of withdrawal." Unnecessary detoxification appears to be a relatively common phenomenon, but it is extremely difficult to estimate just how frequently this might occur. For admittance into those programs that routinely require prior detoxification, it can only be assumed that many patients who might not need detoxification are forced to do so in order that they might meet a given program's admission requirements.

The goals of treatment that programs that are based on the Minnesota Model attempt to achieve have been described as follows:

1. Treatment does not "cure" the disease—the expectation is that by instituting an achievable method of abstinence the disease will be put into remission.
2. All therapeutic efforts are directed at helping the patient reach a level of motivation that will enable him or her to commit to this abstinence program.
3. An educational program is developed to assist the patient in becoming familiar with addictive processes, insight into compulsive behaviors, medical complications, emotional insight, and maintenance of physical, mental, and spiritual health.
4. The patient's family and other significant persons are included in the therapeutic process with the understanding that the therapeutic process does not occur in a vacuum, rather in interpersonal relationships.
5. The patient is indoctrinated into the AA program and instructed as to the content and application of the twelve-step program.
6. Group and individual therapy are directed at self-understanding and acceptance with emphasis on how alcohol and drugs have affected their lives.
7. There is insistence on participation in a longitudinal support and follow-up program based on the belief that, as in the management of all chronic disease processes, maintenance is critically important to the outcome of any therapy. This follow-up usually consists of ongoing support provided by the treatment facility as well as participation in community self-help groups such as AA, Narcotics Anonymous (NA), Opiates Anonymous (OA), and the like (Collins, 1993).

The goals as they are outlined above seem to be reasonable at first glance. But let's translate them into more simple English and see what they are really attempting to accomplish:

1. Convince the patient to believe that he or she suffers from an incurable disease that can only be controlled by abstinence.
2. Get the patient to commit to complete abstinence, forever.
3. Teach the patient that he or she has an incurable disease that causes him or her to crave alcohol or drugs and he or she will crave alcohol or drugs until the day he or she dies.
4. The patient's family is sick too, and they will need to commit to a program that is similar to that which will be prescribed for the patient.
5. Make sure that the patient believes that his or her only hope is to commit to a twelve-step program.
6. Convince the patient that his or her disease is responsible for everything bad that has happened to them.
7. See to it that patient believes that he or she must commit to lifelong participation in therapy and a twelve-step program, or else the chronic disease will kill him or her.

People, this isn't treatment. This really appears more like indoctrination. As Bufe (1998) put it: "It really has little to do with the problem of alcohol abuse. Rather, it's an indoctrination program designed to inculcate both distrust of self and learned helplessness ('powerlessness') in the patient and to convince him that his only hope of salvation is to abandon self-direction and plunge himself into lifelong participation in the religious program of Alcoholics Anonymous—never mind that every single premise upon which this indoctrination is built is demonstrably false."

In a previous chapter, it was pointed out that participation in AA, or in treatment based upon the principles of AA, produces a rate of recovery that is no higher than spontaneous recovery. I, personally, can see no other way to view these goals except to regard them as an overt attempt to sell the ideology that is held so reverently by those who wish to see to it that AA and the twelve-step approach continue to be the only method of treatment that will be made available to those seeking treatment for their addictions, thereby perpetuating the reliance on AA well into the future.

If the points outlined above represent the goals of treatment which have been the mainstay in the treatment of addictions, we probably need to examine exactly how these treatment providers go about accomplishing these goals.

All of the treatment programs based on the twelve-step method attempt only to move the patient through the first four steps of the Twelve Steps that are articulated by AA. These four steps are:

> 1. We admitted that we are powerless over alcohol— that our lives had become unmanageable.
> 2. Came to believe that a power greater than ourselves could restore us to sanity.
> 3. Made a decision to turn our will and our lives over to the care of God as we understood him.
> 4. Made a searching and fearless moral inventory of ourselves. (Alcoholics Anonymous, 1939)

All of the therapy and education offered within these programs is directed toward moving the patient through these four steps. Once this has been achieved, according to the discretion of the program's non-professional counselors, the patient is discharged with the expectation that the patient will continue to work through the remaining steps. Of course, the patient is always reminded that he or she must continue to participate in a twelve-step support group such as AA if he or she is to have any hope of recovering from the disease, and this will likely be necessary for the remainder of his or her life. Very frequently, family members are also strongly encouraged to participate in a twelve-step program as well.

Criticisms of twelve-step treatment have been abundant. In addition to being ineffective and ill-conceived, as has already been demonstrated, twelve-step treatment has also been described as being dogmatic, coercive, and brutal. Some have gone as far as stating that

AA and treatment based on AA is cultlike (Trimpey, 1997; Ragge, 1998).

Claims of this type have frequently been reinforced when former patients of such programs have described their treatment experiences. Peele, Bufe, and Brodsky (2000) offer one patient's account of his experience in a thirty-five-day stay in a Minnesota Model twelve-step treatment facility: "We'd get up in the morning, do calisthenics, eat breakfast, and then go to group therapy, which was basically working the steps. After lunch, we'd have a lecture [in which twelve-step/ disease-concept ideology was presented as established fact], and then after dinner, we'd go to an AA meeting."

While this appears to be a relatively benign description, it certainly serves as an example that such treatment is intended only as indoctrination to AA.

We previously reviewed Dr. Elizabeth Bartlett's account of her experience while placed in a detoxification program. What follows is Dr. Bartlett's description of the treatment she received after she was finally admitted into treatment:

> For anyone who has not been in a 12-step rehab, the daily program is brutal. Mine lasted from 7:30 AM to 10:00 PM. Essentially there was no time to think. If anyone was in his or her room for more than a few minutes, staff went in and announced that "isolating was just going to cause stinking thinking, so get out of your room." Every patient was expected to be at meals exactly on time, and to participate in all scheduled events. Late arrivals resulted in the loss of the minimal telephone contact we were allowed with the outside world. Almost every group, meeting and lecture began with the Serenity Prayer, and ended with the Lord's Prayer.... I was told that "addicts do not like following rules," so many arbitrary rules were imposed to essentially break us of the bad habit of thinking independently. They wanted to break my will, so that I would "snap," and become one of them, obedient and grateful to the program.... I was told

from the moment that I arrived … [that if I] didn't complete their "simple program," there was a 100% chance I would drink again, and would lose my career and my family, and would ultimately die from drinking.… I was not allowed to question anything about AA, especially the religious aspect.… They kept telling me that my thinking was stinking, that my intelligence was a liability and was causing my problems, and that I had better check my psychiatric knowledge at the door and stop thinking. (Bartlett, 1997, pp. 4–5)

Again, what Dr. Bartlett describes appears to be much more of an indoctrination process as opposed to a treatment effort. We can see that such treatment can certainly be perceived as being dogmatic and coercive. Dr. Bartlett described her experience as being a brutal effort to break her will.

Rebecca Fransway's compilation entitled *12-Step Horror Stories* (2000) offers an account of a young woman who attended a "family group" in a treatment facility where her father was being treated for alcoholism:

The facilitator of the group, a man in his thirties I'll call "Rollin," sported a clipboard and intense, quick eyes. I had never been in a therapy group. I did not realize what was happening was *attack therapy* until Rollin and the others began to *attack* people.

He'd start out asking a person how he or she was doing. If she said "fine," or words to that effect, Rollin would say *bullshit!* And then the attack would begin. The word *bullshit* flew about the room quite often, along with defensive explanations, angry diatribes, tears, and much melodrama. I became petrified, because it was apparent that Rollin picked people for group focus out of the blue, and that to say you were okay was the wrong answer. My mind quickly began to search for something I could say was wrong with my life that would be okay to tell these people.

Rollin, and then some of the others, began to yell at one man in particular.

"Bill" had been sent to the VA alcohol program while awaiting sentencing for manslaughter. He had been drinking and driving, and had killed an innocent person. He said he could not remember the accident. *Bullshit!*, Rollin nearly screamed, a lock of brown hair flipping over his eye. *that's pure bullshit! You remember—admit it! You remember everything about that accident—admit it!* Bill's head was hung. Others joined in. I was reminded of the flock of chickens which we had while I grew up. When chickens are under stress, and one of them gets hurt, the rest move in and peck it to death.

I was confused and frightened. I decided I did not know enough about what was going on, so I said nothing. Later my dad told me he didn't think Bill remembered anything about the accident either, but that *attack therapy* consisted of *tough love* designed to crush people's *egos*. It was *big egos*, he said, that stood in the way of alcoholic recovery.

They harangued Bill for quite awhile, then Rollin continued around the room. Folks' personal thoughts, feelings, and lives were pried into, and the accusation *bullshit* flew freely.

I knew this behavior was all wrong, but I didn't know why. Years later, I would understand that my fear and discomfort were correct, healthy emotional responses to the intrusive verbal abuse known in the recovery subculture as *tough love*. In that group, and in many alcoholism/addiction treatment centers, as well as twelve-step groups, people's emotional or ego boundaries are deliberately violated in the name of *tough love.*

I left there with the distinct impression that for all their big talk about *recovery,* such treatment centers provide little more than humiliation for drunks.

According to the young woman who provided the account, she came to believe that what she had observed was nothing less than abuse of the patients that were supposed to be receiving treatment within this particular facility. Fransway's compilation offers many other accounts that are similar to that which is cited here.

As can be seen, there is certainly reason to believe that treatment based on the Minnesota Model can, at times, be dogmatic, coercive, and brutal. When the stated goals of these programs, along with the prescribed method of achieving these goals, are examined, it becomes very clear that what is offered in the name of treatment is nothing more than an organized and intensified effort to indoctrinate people to the beliefs and practices of AA. Since nothing but the twelve-step method is offered within these programs, it all but guarantees that patients will depart from these treatment programs believing their only hope for salvation is dependent entirely upon their continued reliance on twelve-step support groups such as AA, NA, and so on.

Is twelve-step treatment actually cultlike indoctrination? Some have articulated the belief that this is so. Jack Trimpey, in an article entitled "Alcoholics Anonymous: Of Course It's a Cult!" (1997) stated the following:

For the record, here is our position: *Of course AA is a cult!* AA is not only a religious cult, it is a radical cult, an evil cult, a widespread cult, and a dangerous cult. AA has become an engine of social decay posing as a noble, altruistic fellowship. Its perverse philosophy of sin-disease and deliverance by faith in a heterogeneous deity contradicts the fundamental values of a free society, but is uniquely appealing to people addicted to substance-pleasure. AA is a cancer on the soul of the nation, producing no pain to the populace as it eats away at the foundation of society. Its victims are its members who become grateful to their captors. AA is causing the problem it says it helps. Its twelve-step program suggests nothing on how to quit an addiction except to stop trying, and its members love the cult more than any newcomer. Each cult member shares a vision of a better world resulting from propagating the steps—not from the effects of abstinence upon society. The AA cult has infiltrated our federal and state bureaucracies and now nests in every social institution, setting policies that funnel new members into its craw. It expands for its own sake and cannot change from within. Therefore, it must be destroyed by forthright public education and exposé.

Obviously, Jack Trimpey feels strongly that AA is a cult in every sense of the word.

In *Alcoholics Anonymous: Cult or Cure* (1998), author Charles Bufe analyzed the characteristics of AA against twenty-three criteria which he believed were defining in making a determination as to whether or not an organizational entity could be determined to be a cult. Bufe concluded that AA could be considered to be "cult-lite" in that it could definitely be associated with sixteen of the twenty-three qualifying criteria. While falling short of declaring AA to be a full-fledged cult, Bufe did offer this opinion in his closing comments:

> Finally, it's worth noting that while brazenly destructive cults such as the People's Temple and Heaven's Gate have considerably worse effects upon their individual members than AA has upon its individual members, the commonly cited religious cults have very limited numbers of followers (despite self-serving gross overestimates) and have very little

influence in society at large, while AA is a mass organization with a very extensive hidden structure that has *tremendous* influence in society. Thus, it could well be that AA does more harm to society— and to far greater numbers of people—than all other religious cults combined (Chapter 10).

Micheal Langone (1998) offered these criteria in defining cults that utilize thought reform (mind control) programs:

1. Obtaining substantial control over an individual's time and thought content, typically by gaining control over major elements of the person's social and physical environment;
2. Systematically creating a sense of powerlessness in the person;
3. Manipulating a system of rewards, punishments, and experiences in such a way as to promote new learning of an ideology or belief system/behavior advocated by leadership;
4. Maintaining a closed system of logic and an authoritarian structure in the organization;
5. Maintaining a noninformed state existing in the subject.
   (p. 3)

While Dr. Langone made no mention of these criteria in comparison to AA, it would be relatively easy to make a case that suggests that AA does, in many respects, conform to these defining characteristics.

Making a determination as to whether or not AA is a cult is not an intended objective of this effort. The mere fact that AA has been compared to a cult indicates there is much about this organization which warrants serious scrutiny. What does seem brazenly apparent is that twelve-step treatment programs do appear to have indoctrination into AA as the primary goal of treatment. Since neither AA nor twelve-step treatment has ever demonstrated that adherence to AA ideology is effective in battling addictions, one can only wonder as to why it has, and continues to be, the mainstay of treatment in this nation.

At this point, the reader might be asking: is the treatment being offered in more than 90 percent of our nation's treatment programs really as bad and as nefarious as that which is being described? My personal response to such a question would have to be: yes, it can certainly be that bad in some instances. It can actually be much more abusive and vicious than has been portrayed in the few accounts that have been provided herein. I would offer this response based on my observations that have come from working in and around the addictions treatment industry for nearly twenty years. I also offer my response based upon my experience of having been the recipient of such treatment.

I can state that I have witnessed that addiction counselors do frequently engage brutal and vicious verbal attacks on their patients in order to "help" them to overcome their "denial." Addictions counselors usually, in an effort to break through the denial or some other perceived obstacle presented by the patient, engage in a group-therapy technique that is unique to addictions treatment. This technique has frequently been referred to as the "hot seat." Each member of the treatment group will eventually get a turn at sitting on the hot seat. Some get more than one turn according to whether or not the counselor feels that the patient is still holding on to some thread of self-reliance.

When a patient is selected for his or her turn on the hot seat, the verbal assault usually begins with the counselor confronting the patient on some issue or behavior that they believe is causing the patient to remain, as they call it, stuck. Then, each member of the group is allowed and encouraged to confront the selected patient. It is not at all unusual for this confrontation to become intensely personal and extremely ferocious. I have been witness to endless badgering of patients to the point that the patients would be willing to admit to almost anything in order to end the harassment to which they are being subjected to, regardless of whether that admission would be true or false. I have witnessed behavior on the part of treatment professionals that has left me feeling ashamed to admit that I have ever had any association with the addiction treatment industry.

I can't honestly state that I know that this type of maltreatment exists in all the treatment facilities utilizing the twelve-step method. It would be my sincere hope that such treatment would represent the exception and not the rule. Unfortunately, there exist far too many reports of this type of maltreatment for us to assume that such behavior occurs only as isolated instances. When it is realized that treatment based on twelve-step ideology really does represent more of an indoctrination process as opposed to any real attempt to actually treat a problem, it becomes very easy to visualize the possibility that some practitioners in this indoctrination effort might become overenthused in their efforts to convince patients that they must conform to this ideology. Unfortunately, for those who have paid dearly for the privilege of receiving treatment for their addictions, what they are actually getting when they are subjected to this harassing form of treatment represents not only a violation of ethical practices, but it also represents a violation of their individual rights. In my mind, any activity that is to be pursued in an effort to provide therapy can neither violate ethical standards nor the patients' rights. If it does, it's not therapy.

What has definitely occurred to me as a result of the experiences I have accumulated within this field is that programs which base their treatment efforts on twelve-step ideologies are doomed to failure. As one truly begins to examine the belief system that has been advanced by AA and its ever-persistent promoters, it becomes very clear that the logic upon which this system of beliefs is based simply makes the kind of sense that is (to use popular vernacular) NOT! It is a mistaken set of beliefs from the outset.

Initially, we have the creation of a concept that asserted that alcoholism is a disease. AA (1939) viewed alcoholism as being a "manifestation of an allergy" (p. xxviii). The alcoholic was, therefore, "bodily and mentally different" from other human beings, and he or she suffered from a 'progressive illness' which only got worse, never better" (p. 30).

The concept was expanded over the years until alcoholism evolved into a primary, chronic disease that has its origins in our genetic makeup. This is the more modern terminology used by AA's biggest promoter NCADD. It must be reiterated that the evolution of this concept, and the subsequent promotion of the concept, occurred in the complete absence of any scientific evidence that could support such a conceptualization with regard to alcoholism or addiction to any other substance.

Even though we know that this conceptualization is demonstrably false, let us, for a moment, pretend that it is true. Let's pretend that addiction is a disease that is progressive, incurable, and frequently fatal if left untreated. Obviously, we don't want to see people suffer or die from this disease over which the victim has no control. We must, therefore, find a medical cure for this disease, or at the very least, a medical treatment that will control the disease.

Well, medical science didn't have a cure for the disease, as Dr. Silkworth pointed out in the Big Book (p. xxviii). Never fear, Dr. Bob and Bill W. came up with a reliable and effective treatment for the disease. They called it the "Twelve Steps," and if the addicted person follows these twelve simple steps he or she will be relieved of this disease. Wait! It's not a medical treatment, it's a spiritual treatment. Alas, we now have the very first, and the only, spiritual treatment for a medical disease.

There has never been anything like this before, nor has there ever been anything like it since. It's such a revelation, a veritable miracle of a treatment. We must institute this treatment all throughout the land. We must treat all people who suffer from this disease by this miraculous method.

Of course, since this treatment is such a miracle, we had better charge everybody plenty for the application of this miracle, maybe as much as forty-seven thousand dollars per person. Since Dr. Bob only used the first four of these twelve wonderful steps when he treated alcoholics in Akron, Ohio, we only need to do the same. It should take exactly twenty-eight days for these diseased individuals to master these first four miraculous steps. That should put them well on their way to a much brighter future. Of course, they must be willing to go on and finish the remaining eight steps in AA, NA, or some other twelve-step program if they are to be fully vested in the brightest future possible. That ought to keep those little devils busy for the rest of their lives.

And, hey, we don't even have to employ professional therapists to assist these diseased individuals in getting through these first four steps. We can simply have recovering alcoholics and drug addicts help them along their way. That's what Bill W. and Dr. Bob did. After all, they're in recovery and they've been through it all. They know exactly how to show the diseased individual how to approach the steps in just the right way.

Okay then, that seems to work out nicely. We have realized that addiction, in all its forms, is a disease. We can effectively treat it with the first four steps of the Twelve Steps of Alcoholics Anonymous. We know this because seventy years of experience in doing it this way proves it so. However, just to make sure, perhaps we should take a closer look at these four steps and see what they really accomplish.

> *Step One.* We admitted that we were powerless over alcohol, that our lives had become unmanageable.

In this step, the addicted person learns that he or she rests at the mercy of the greater power of alcohol or other drugs. The addicted person also learns that he or she has absolutely no control over any aspect of his or her life because he or she is powerless. The addicted person learns that he or she is no longer an "I"; he or she becomes a part of the "we"—part of the group. This alleviates any need for the addicted person to assume any responsibility for himself or herself. The individual becomes part of the "we" who, as mere individuals, also have no power.

> *Step Two.* We came to believe that a Power greater than ourselves could restore us to Sanity.

In the second step, the addicted person, who is now just a part of the "we," learns that his or her only hope for change resides in a power that is outside of him or her. The addicted person also learns that, not only is he or she addicted, he or she is now insane as well. The individual is now dependent upon the power to restore his or her sanity and sobriety.

> *Step Three.* We made a decision to turn our will and our lives over to the care of God as we understood him.

In the third step, the addicted person, having accepted that he or she is powerless, insane, and no longer has any identity of his or her own, must now decide to sit and wait for some sane and powerful force outside himself or herself to take control of his or her existence. Although, the term "God" implies a Christian conceptualization of God, this cannot be. Anyone who understands Christianity readily accepts that God's spirit resides in every individual. That is to say, the individual is not separate from God; the individual is part of God. According to the Big Book (p.60), "any life run on self-will can hardly be a success." Again, this is contrary to the Christian concept of free will. The Big Book, in the chapter entitled "We Agnostics" (pp. 44–57), discusses the concept of God extensively. It is clear from what is being stated therein that any sense of God's spirit must come from outside oneself.

> *Step Four.* We made a searching and fearless moral inventory of ourselves.

The Big Book states that the purpose of this is to "disclose damaged or unsalable goods, to get rid of them without regret" (p. 64). However, it is easy to see that among the messages that might be imparted in this step is more to the effect that the addict has undesirable characteristics that makes him or her "no good"; that there is something about the individual which sets him or her apart from others who have "good" characteristics. If the addict cannot rid him or herself of those characteristics, or defects, he or she is a failure and is unacceptable. The only place where the addict might find acceptance is within the group: the "we." This is a step that can lead to a rejection of self, or it can cause the addict to lapse into unbearable feelings of guilt and shame.

This, purely and simply, is indoctrination. When closely examining the treatment that is provided in programs based on the twelve-step model, the only conclusion that becomes evident is that this model cannot be considered to be anything other than an indoctrination process. All that is attempted in the name of education and therapy is directed toward engendering an acceptance of the disease concept as it is promoted by AA; convincing that patient that he or she must commit to lifelong abstinence; and convincing the patient that his or her only hope for salvation lies in his or her willingness to surrender himself or herself to lifelong devotion to the twelve steps as promoted by AA.

These steps cannot, by any understandable definition, be considered a treatment for anything. What these steps ask an individual to do is absolutely contrary to any ethical, moral, and legal approach to the treatment any of other disorder known to man.

Goals of treatment that can be considered as being ethical, moral, and legal would include: 1) acceptance of personal responsibility; 2) individual empowerment; 3) self-determination; 4) self-direction; 5) self-acceptance; 6) personal independence; 7) development of internal resources; and 8) facilitation of spiritual awakening, placing faith in the individual's ability to heal and grow.

As can be seen upon examination of the four steps used in the treatment of addictions in more than 90 percent of all of the treatment programs that currently exist, this method of treatment can only be considered to be antithetical to what is considered to be ethical, moral, and legal treatment in any other clinical context.

What is truly sad is that, according to SAMSHA (1997), roughly 270,000 individuals were coerced into twelve-step treatment programs by the judicial and penal systems during the year 1995. Many others are coerced into twelve-step treatment through Employee Assistance Programs (EAPs) and professional diversion programs that exist within the medical, legal, and a variety of other professions. This means that multitudes of individuals have literally been forced to endure treatment that is, at the very least, contrary in practice to the ethical and moral standards that would be expected relative to the treatment of any other illness or disorder. This might be justifiable in some sense if such treatment worked. Clearly, it does not. Clearly, it cannot.

The evidence provided thus far in this effort should clearly demonstrate the twelve-step ideology that has been promoted by AA and its ever persistent supporters has never actually delivered on their promise of a better future. Most people who have been treated in twelve-step programs fail in their efforts to overcome their problems with addiction. Membership in AA, at best, can claim a success rate of only 5 percent.

Our collective reliance on this ill-conceived ideology, with its failed method of treating addictions, has been imprudent, to say the least. Substance use problems in this nation have steadily increased, showing no signs that any hope of improvement lies ahead. Those individuals who received treatment guided by twelve-step doctrine have, by all reasonable estimates, relapsed and continued to abuse alcohol and drugs approximately 95 percent of the time. Even repeated exposure to this type of treatment appears to have little or no effect. Twelve-step treatment has been exposed in terms of its efficacy. Additionally, it has been demonstrated that such treatment is very costly, and it has been shown to be ethically and morally, and even legally, questionable in some instances.

Knowing all of this, how can anyone continue to support the notion that twelve-step ideology should continue to be supported as a viable means of treating addictions? To do so can only be considered to be misanthropic.

While I don't necessarily agree with Jack Trimpey's assertion that AA is a cult, I do emphatically agree with his assertion that AA and the ideology which it attempts to promote "has infiltrated our federal and state bureaucracies and now nests in every social institution, setting policies that funnel new members into its craw. It expands for its own sake, and cannot change from within. Therefore, it must be destroyed by forthright public education and exposé."

References

Chapter Five

Alcoholics Anonymous. (1939). *The Story of How More than One Hundred Men Have Recovered from Alcoholism. Fourth Edition (2001).* Works Publishing Company.

Alcoholics Anonymous. (1980). *Dr. Bob and the Good Oldtimers.* (pp. 82–83). New York, NY: Alcoholics Anonymous World Services, Inc.

Alcoholics Anonymous. (1989). *Alcoholics Anonymous Comes of Age.* Written by Bill Wilson. (p. viii). New York: Alcoholics Anonymous World Services Inc.

Anderson, D. J., McGovern, J. P., and DuPont, R. L. (1999). The origins of the Minnesota model of addiction—A first person account. American Society of Addiction Medicine. *Journal of Addictive Disease,* **18(4).**

Bartlett, E. (1997). Brainwashing 101, or how I survived 12-step rehab. *Journal of Rational Recovery,* **10(1),** 4.

Bufe, C. (1998). *Alcoholics Anonymous: Cult or Cure.* 2nd edition, revised. San Francisco, CA: See Sharp Press.

Collins, G. B. (1993). Contemporary issues in the treatment of alcohol dependence. *Psychiatric Clinics of North America,* **16(1),** 35.

Fransway, R. (2000). *12-Step Horror Stories: True Tales of Misery, Betrayal, and Abuse in NA, AA, and 12-Step Treatment.* (63–67). Tucson, AZ: See Sharp Press.

Hazelden Foundation. (1994). The Hazelden Report entitled "Minnesota model began as an effort in social reform." Originally printed in the Nov. 1, 1994 edition of the *Star Tribune*. Web site: http://www.hazelden.org.

Hazelden Foundation (2004). Web site: http://www.hazelden.org.

Langone, M. D. (Ed.). (1998). *Recovery from Cults*. New York, NY: W.W. Norton & Company.

Nace, E. P. (1993). Impatient treatment. Marc Galanter, (Ed.), *Recent Developments in Alcoholism*, (Volume 11, p. 430).

Peele, S., Bufe, C., and Brodsky, A. (2000). *Resisting 12-Step Coercion: How to Fight Participation in AA, NA or 12-Step Treatment*. Tucson, AZ: See Sharp Press.

Ragge, K. (1998). *The Real AA: Behind the Myth of 12-step Recovery*. Tucson, AZ: See Sharp Press.

Roman, P., and Blum, T. (1997). *National Treatment Summary Report*. (p. 20). Athens, GA: Institute for Behavioral Research.

Schmidt, L., and Weisner, C. (1993). Developments in alcoholism treatment. Marc Galanter, (Ed.), *Recent Developments in Alcoholism*. (Volume 11, p. 378).

Substance Abuse and Mental Health Services Administration. (1997). *National Admissions to Substance Abuse Treatment Services: The Treatment Episode Data Set (TEDS) 1992–1995*. Rockville, Maryland. (Table 11, p. 47; Table 10, p. 46).

Trimpey, J. (1997). Alcoholics anonymous: Of course it's a cult. *Journal of Rational Recovery*, **9(5).**

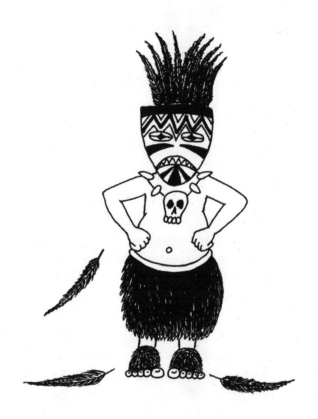

Chapter Six

Misfeasance: Unqualified People
Doing Very Bad Things.

In the previous chapter, I made several references to the fact the treatment provided by programs that utilize the Minnesota Model, or the twelve-step approach, is often delivered by non-professional counselors. This is, in fact, considered to be a key element of the Minnesota Model. It was written, "The key element of this approach to addiction treatment was the blending of professional and trained nonprofessional (recovering) staff around the principles of Alcoholics Anonymous" (Anderson, et al., 1999). In describing the model it is also stated, "There was an individualized treatment plan (Ibid)." As it appears to be the case with so many things that have been found to be true of treatment based on this model, these two elements which are considered to be key characteristics of the model may not be truly representative of what is actually practiced in programs that implement this model. When closely examined, what is actually put into practice in many of the treatment programs based on this model can certainly be considered to be questionable in relation to the ethical and legal standards that are common to most of the helping professions. Such an examination will also exemplify how AA doctrine has become so deeply embedded within the addiction treatment industry that it may be very difficult, or at least very problematic, to bring about needed changes within the treatment industry.

The first key element that we will examine is that of the development and implementation of "individualized treatment plans."

In most states, there exist minimal standards established to guide the development of alcohol and drug treatment programs within a given state. In order for any treatment facility or program to be legally licensed, it must demonstrate that the treatment offered meets or exceeds these minimal standards. Licensing authorities in many states require that an individualized treatment plan will be created for each individual admitted for treatment in a licensed treatment facility. Most often, it is required that this should be a plan that represents a collaborative effort between the patient and the patient's counselor. The patient is often required to sign the treatment plan as an indication that he or she has participated in its creation and that he or she approves of and accepts the treatment plan that is to be implemented.

Treatment plans are generally considered to be a specific road map to the treatment that will be provided to a patient. Treatment plans, in general, must list the patient's primary problem(s) and then outline specific goals and objectives to be achieved in order to assist the patient in overcoming his or her problem(s). Goals and objectives should, as much as possible, be stated in concrete and measurable terms. In many instances, treatment plans must be reviewed over specified intervals of time in order to assess the progress that is being made toward attainment of the goals and objectives. Any treatment activity directed toward assisting a given patient in his or her efforts to make progress toward accomplishing specific objectives, or toward attaining specific goals, should also be documented in such a way that the association between the activity and the treatment goals and objectives is clearly evident.

It would be reasonable to assume that in treatment programs designed to treat substance use disorders, there would exist some homogeneity in the goals and objectives stated in each patient's treatment plan. For example, a major goal that might be common to each of the patients in a given treatment program would be that of achieving an ongoing state of abstinence, since that is apparently the primary goal of most twelve-step treatment programs. However, it would also be reasonable to assume the treatment plans would also vary from patient to patient in order to address the unique problems which might be presented by any given patient.

Keeping this in mind and knowing that almost all treatment programs based on the Minnesota Model strive to achieve the same goals for each of their patients, and that they attempt to accomplish these goals simply by moving the client through the first four of the Twelve Steps of AA, it becomes very apparent that the notion of an individualized treatment plan is a virtual impossibility.

Let us look at an example. Let's assume that one of the goals of treatment for a given patient would be to overcome denial. According to AA doctrine, the first step of the Twelve Steps relates to the issue of denial. That is, once the patient completes his or her first step, he or she will have admitted that he or she has an alcohol or drug problem. So, we end up with a goal/objective statement that appears as follows:

Goal 1.   Objective 1.
Overcome denial   *The patient will complete the first step.*

On the surface, this appears to make some sense. The goal is stated in somewhat concrete and measurable terms. But, the objective is not. How do we know if, how, or when the patient might accomplish this objective? Does the objective even directly relate to the goal?

It will be recalled that that the first step states, "We admitted that we were powerless over alcohol, that our lives had become unmanageable." Do admissions of powerless and unmanageability equate to an acknowledgement and identification of the patient's problem? When a patient completes this step, has the patient acknowledged that he or she is experiencing a specific problem and is accepting of some ownership of his or her behavior? On the other hand, does the completion of this step actually take the patient a step in the opposite direction?

Here, what is actually occurring is that the patient is assigning the problem to "we" as opposed to the patient actually stating "I." This does not constitute an acceptance of personal ownership of a problem. Also, the patient is stating that he or she rests at the mercy of the greater power of alcohol or other drugs. It has taken control of the patient despite valiant efforts to remain in control of life. The patient is stating that he or she has absolutely no control over any aspect of life because he or she has been rendered powerless by alcohol. The patient is stating that he or she is a victim of alcohol. The patient learns that he or she is no longer an "I"; he or she becomes a part of the "we"; part of the collective group. This alleviates any need for the person to assume any personal responsibility for himself or herself. The patient simply becomes part of the "we" who, outside of the collective, no longer has personal relevance.

Attainment of the goal of overcoming denial would render it necessary that the person admits that he or she, individually, has a specific problem. Such an admission on the part of the patient would indicate the acceptance of some responsibility for and ownership of the problem. But, this is not what is stated in this first step, nor is it what is intended to be accomplished in this step.

In reality, the objective does nothing in regard to empowering or encouraging the patient to attain the goal that is stated. In fact, it actually encourages the patient to abandon personal responsibility and ownership of the problem. It encourages the patient to assume that he or she is powerless and is completely incapable of managing life. He or she must surrender themselves to the "we" in order to find salvation.

Believe it or not, I have frequently seen treatment plans that include goal/objective statements exactly like that which I have used as an example. This is not a legitimate way to plan for treatment. This cannot, by any stretch of the imagination, even be considered to be treatment. This would not be considered to be a legitimate or an effective way to plan for the treatment of any other mental disorder. No wonder it doesn't work!

I can recall that, one time in the past, I reviewed a treatment plan that had been created for an individual who was determined to be suffering from depression. This patient's treatment plan included the goal/objective statement as follows:

Goal	Objective
Alleviate depression.	*Untie the patient's internal knots.*

Obviously, this couldn't be considered to be a realistic or legitimate treatment plan. The therapist who devised this plan was instructed to create a real treatment plan that would outline what specific strategies would need to be implemented in order for the patient to engage in a realistic effort directed toward overcoming depression. The strategies had to be stated in concrete and measurable terms, and there would have to be a clear association between the strategies that would be recommended and the goal that would be attained.

As ridiculous as the above goal/objective statement appears to be, it is no more ridiculous than what is contained within the treatment plans frequently utilized in the twelve-step treatment programs that exist in all fifty states within our nation. When you carefully examine the goals and objectives of twelve-step treatment of addictions, you can see that there is no real way a treatment effort based on the first four steps of AA can address the individual needs of any patient. Traditional twelve-step efforts totally ignore the notion of individuality. There is no "I" in twelve-step treatment. The twelve-step method is universally applied to all addicted persons, regardless of their individual problems or circumstances. It is a "one method cures all ills" approach. This is just one of the reasons that the twelve-step approach cannot be considered to be a legitimate method of treating any disorder.

In today's addiction treatment industry, devising and implementing treatment plans similar to that which was exemplified is considered to be acceptable. In as much as 90 percent of all treatment programs in this nation fully endorse and follow the twelve-step model, it appears as though planning treatment in this manner is not only acceptable, it is preferred. This serves as an indication as to how firmly entrenched AA doctrine has become not only within those who offer such treatment, but also in those who administer these treatment programs; and they set the standards for addictions treatment. Bufe (1998) stated:

> Because they've been thoroughly indoctrinated into the AA/disease concept belief system, these facts matter not at all to those administering and conducting twelve-step treatment programs. For them, having turned their lives and will over to God, The Program has become a matter of faith; and even to question the

premises of their belief system is blasphemous. They know "The Truth"—as revealed by Bill Wilson in the "inspired" Big Book. As well, they believe that their sobriety and their very lives depend on "carrying this message to those not yet saved," so they often carry that message with fearful zeal.

So, the treatment of addictions in our nation is guided not by the implementation of realistic, concrete, and measurable individualized treatment planning, but it is guided by faith—"The Truth" as revealed in the Big Book.

The sad truth of the matter is that many of those charged with the responsibility of treating addicted persons within this nation are so fully indoctrinated in AA ideology, and little else, that they are truly incapable of approaching treatment of addictions in any other way. For the most part, counselors in the addiction treatment industry are not qualified to treat anything beyond addiction. It is, therefore, questionable as to whether or not they are qualified even to treat addictions. Certified or licensed chemical dependency counselors, as a whole, are largely uneducated in terms of their overall understanding of human behavior, and they are not fully trained in any discipline that would provide them with the clinical skills that would prepare them to be able to accurately diagnose or to treat any mental disorder. For some, their primary qualification as a counselor is that they found their own recovery in a twelve-step program, and they wish to carry on that message.

At the outset of this chapter, reference was made to the fact that one of the key elements in the Minnesota Model was that of the "blending of professional and trained nonprofessional (recovering) staff around the principles of Alcoholics Anonymous" (Anderson, et al., 1999). It must be suggested that the term "blending" may be an overstatement. Yes, there are some persons that practice within the addictions treatment industry who are qualified professionals and are credentialed in such disciplines as medicine, psychology, counseling, or social work. These qualified credentialed professionals truly do represent a minority in terms of those who actually provide the day-to-day treatment of addictions. Most of the addictions counselors who provide the online treatment in twelve-step programs do not possess such professional qualifications. The overwhelming majority of these counselors are either certified or licensed chemical dependency counselors. Despite the fact that these so-called counselors may be licensed or certified by some authority, does not necessarily mean they are even reasonably qualified to conduct or provide treatment services that have any realistic chance of helping their patients.

In the earlier days of treatment, there existed a great deal of variability from one state to another as to what would qualify an individual to become an addictions counselor. In some states, all that was required was that the candidate could demonstrate the achievement of a specified period of sobriety, sometimes as little as six months, and that he or she received some training in a formal treatment program. Sometimes, only six weeks of hands-on training was required before the potential addictions counselor was able to work without direct supervision. The only qualification that is required according to AA doctrine is that of membership in AA.

When insurance companies began to pay for addiction treatment in the 1970s, there was some insistence that addictions counselors should be, in some way, qualified to provide such treatment. In the present day, most insurance companies will not reimburse for inpatient treatment unless that treatment is supervised by a physician or another qualified credentialed professional. This insistence on the part of the insurance industry motivated many states to establish minimum standards for the credentialing of addictions counselors. When states did begin to establish minimal qualifications for certification as addictions counselors, many who had been practicing within the industry, as it had evolved to that point in time, were simply grandfathered. That is, they were issued certification or licensure simply because they already practiced within the industry.

Even today, however, the minimum standards that are required of addictions counselors do not begin to compare to the credentialing requirements for other professionals who are considered to be qualified to treat any other mental disorder.

The National Association of Alcohol and Drug Abuse Counselors (NAADAC) is the largest national organization that represents the interests of substance abuse counselors. The organization boasts a membership of more than twelve thousand persons and they have state affiliate associations in forty-six of the fifty states. NAADAC also offers several levels of certification of counselors ranging from entry level counselors (level one) to what they call "Master Addiction Counselor." Listed are the qualifications that NAADAC requires for level one certification:

- Current state certification/licensure as an alcoholism and/or drug-abuse counselor
- Three years fulltime or six thousand hours of supervised experience as an alcoholism and/or drug abuse counselor
- Two-hundred seventy contact hours of education and training in alcoholism and drug abuse or related counseling subjects
- A passing score on the national examination for Level 1. (NAADAC, 2005)

These requirements match, and sometimes exceed, most states' requirements for certification or licensure as a substance abuse counselor.

For convenience, I will cite the requirements for my home state, Nebraska, to outline what many states require in terms of qualifications for certification or licensure as a substance abuse counselor. I have found that minimum requirements for most states are comparable. In order to become an alcohol/drug abuse counselor in Nebraska, a person must fulfill the following requirements (State of Nebraska, 1998):

1. High school diploma or GED.
2. Two-hundred seventy contact hours of education in the following areas: forty-five hours of Counseling Theories and Techniques of Casework; forty-five hours Group Counseling; thirty hours of Human Growth and Development; fifteen hours of Professional Ethics and Issues Coursework; thirty hours of Alcohol/Drug Assessment; thirty hours of Multicultural Counseling;

forty-five hours in Medical and Psychosocial Aspects of Alcohol/Drug Use; thirty hours of Clinical Treatment Issues in Chemical Dependency Coursework.

3. Three hundred hours of supervised training in a work setting where alcohol/drug treatment counseling is provided.

4. Six thousand hours of clinically supervised work experience providing alcohol/drug treatment counseling services to alcohol and other drug clients for remuneration.

5. Submission of three letters of reference from persons credentialed in the addictions treatment field.

6. Passage of written and oral examinations to demonstrate competencies.

Substitution of a college degree in counseling, addictions, psychology, social work, or sociology can be made for clinically supervised work experience; two thousand hours for a bachelor's degree; four thousand hours for a master's degree (Ibid.).

At first glance, it would seem that it takes quite a bit of preparation to become a certified alcohol and drug abuse counselor. But, let's look a bit closer at these requirements. First, it appears as if the only real educational requirement is that a potential alcohol and drug counselor must have graduated from high school or obtained an equivalency diploma.

Second, the two-hundred seventy hours of education, as outlined, do not need to be college courses; only courses or training seminars that have been approved by the certifying authority. The two-hundred seventy hours of education required is in the form of contact hours. Roughly, it takes approximately fifteen contact hours to equate to one college credit. Therefore, the education required to be provisionally certified as a counselor that is qualified to provide alcohol and drug treatment services is roughly equivalent to eighteen to twenty credit hours of college education, or the equivalent of approximately six or seven college classes.

Most accredited colleges require somewhere in the vicinity of one-hundred twenty five credit hours in order to graduate with a bachelor's degree in any discipline. At least thirty-two hours of those one-hundred twenty five credits must be from an individual's major field of study. For example, the University of Nebraska at Kearney (1999) requires a total of one-hundred twenty five credits hours in order to graduate with a Bachelor of Science degree. If that degree is with a major in psychology, thirty-six credit hours must be in psychology as required by that department, and twenty-four credit hours must be in a minor area of study.

It is very easy to see that the education required in order to be eligible for certification as an alcohol and drug counselor does not even come close to an undergraduate degree in any discipline.

A counselor must have six thousand hours, or three years full-time supervised experience in the provision of treatment services to be eligible for certification. If you consider that more than 90 percent of treatment programs utilize the twelve-step approach, guess what kind of experience a potential counselor is going to get during that period of time? If you guessed six thousand hours of twelve-step treatment, you would have at least a 90 percent chance of being correct. In Nebraska, that percentage would be much higher.

The question is, for what other mental disorder would we presume that a person who has taken the equivalent of only six or seven college classes, and has three years of exposure to only one approach to treating any disorder, would be qualified to provide effective treatment? The correct answer is none! Under any other circumstance, for any other mental disorder, the minimum educational requirement which is considered an adequate level of preparation to be able to offer treatment for any other mental disorder is that of a master's degree in a behavioral science such as psychology, counseling, social work, or nursing.

During my time as a director of an alcohol and drug treatment facility, I have had the opportunity to supervise many alcohol and drug counselors. Some of those that I supervised had obtained college degrees prior to becoming certified or licensed as alcohol and drug counselors; some had not. I will tell you, without any reservations, there is a distinct and vivid difference between those individuals who saw fit to acquire a formal education compared to those who did not. Those who were formally educated consistently demonstrated a higher degree of professionalism. The more educated persons were much more disciplined in all their efforts and had many more clinical skills which they could put into practice. Overall, they were consistently much more effective compared to those counselors who had not obtained a degree in a behavioral discipline.

In the very first treatment program which I designed and implemented, the program started out with four counselors. Two of the counselors had bachelor degrees in the behavioral sciences. One of those had started working toward a master's degree. Neither of these two counselors was a recovering alcoholic or addict. Both had obtained the chemical dependency counseling licenses. The remaining two were both recovering individuals who had obtained their licenses by following a training program that was stipulated by the state's chemical dependency counselor licensing authority that demanded the two-hundred seventy hours of education, three years experience, etc. Neither of these two counselors had college degrees. One of these counselors had been trained at Hazelden and was certified by NAADAC as a level one counselor. The latter two counselors had previously worked in only twelve-step treatment programs.

This was a treatment program that was started from scratch. As such, there was a period of approximately six months wherein the program could not offer treatment to anyone, pending approval of the program's licensing. During this period, all program counselors and other support staff were given training on a variety of relevant topics that included diagnosis and treatment planning, implementation of various approaches to treating addictions, case management, etc. The program was not designed nor intended to be a twelve-step treatment program.

When the program began to actually treat addicted persons, it became very clear that all of the four counselors had been fully indoctrinated into the twelve-step approach. All four counselors experienced some problems in approaching treatment from a perspective that did not include having the patients follow the first four of the twelve steps. Both of the two counselors that did not have the benefit of a college degree were absolutely lost. Literally, these two counselors had no other foundation of knowledge or experience to draw from except twelve-step treatment. Fortunately, they were willing to learn. The two counselors who had obtained college degrees faired much better in terms of adjusting to different approaches because they did have some familiarity with the theoretical foundations upon which other approaches could be based.

Comparing the relative preparedness between these two sets of counselors was like comparing night and day. The contrast between the two sets was stark to say the least.

The non-degreed counselors literally had to be started from zero. Neither of these counselors had ever even seen a diagnostic and statistical manual (DSM). They could not accurately diagnose their patients' problems because they did not know how to classify their patients' symptoms in a systematic or disciplined manner. These counselors could not even write coherent treatment plans. Because they could not plan their treatment, they had no way of approaching their patients' problems in any other way except to loosely base their efforts on the Twelve Steps.

The two non-degreed counselors did not know how to conduct therapeutic group counseling sessions, despite the fact that they had been doing groups in other programs for several years. I recall that one had complained that he did not feel that he was making any progress within his group of patients during group counseling sessions. In response to that complaint, I asked all counselors to videotape their group sessions. Patients, of course, were asked to sign written releases to allow us to do this.

When I reviewed these tapes with the non-degreed counselors, it was apparent that all each counselor knew how to do was to conduct "mini-AA meetings" in their groups. That is, they spent much of their time going from patient to patient, having each patient recite his or her stories. Everybody in the group sat wherever he or she wanted to while sipping their coffee and cokes. We did not allow smoking in the facility; otherwise patients would have been smoking in group as well. In essence, it was very clear that neither of these counselors had any clue as to how to conduct group therapy. These counselors did not know how to conduct individual therapy either. All that they could effectively accomplish with their patients individually was to offer them guidance in following the Steps.

The two degreed counselors also had some problems in adjusting to other approaches of treating their patients. However, because they had been educated to approach problems in a systematic and disciplined manner, and because they did understand human behavior to a much greater extent, this set of counselors had far less difficulty in learning what they needed to do in order to effectively deal with the problems their patients presented to them.

Obviously, my time during the first year of the program's operation was spent in simply teaching counselors how to do treatment. They all knew how to do twelve-step treatment, but that was all that any of them had ever been exposed to in terms of offering treatment for addictions. Fortunately, all four of the counselors were open to new learning, and they were willing to try different ways of treating addictions. Over time, they all learned to be effective.

My purpose in telling of these experiences is simply to illustrate that many counselors working in the treatment industry know only one way to treat addictions, the twelve-step method. Though each of these four counselors were licensed, meaning each of them had at least three years of experience in treating addictions, none of the four knew any other way to do treatment.

My purpose is also to illustrate that those counselors who do not have any formal training in the behavioral sciences generally do not have a sufficient educational foundation from which they can easily develop the clinical skills they need to become effective in treating addictions. Two hundred and seventy contact hours of education does very little to prepare a prospective counselor for the challenges that he or she will face as he or she begins to attempt to treat addicted persons.

The treatment program described eventually grew. It also became a state-approved counselor training institution. Over the years that I directed this program, I also supervised the training of many chemical dependency counselors in terms of offering them the experience they needed to become licensed. What I consistently observed was that those counselors whose education consisted only of the two-hundred seventy hours required by the state authority were wholly unprepared to function as counselors. They lacked any form of professional discipline. They had very little education with regard to behavioral theory. They had no basis for the development of clinical skills. They completely lacked any formal education in empirical science. As such knowledge was lacking, they did not even have the ability to understand the scientific literature that existed within the addictions treatment field, nor did they understand diagnostic testing.

Counselors that did have at least a bachelor's degree in one of the behavioral sciences had a distinct advantage because they had been required to become disciplined, they did have a general understanding of human behavior, and they could more readily build upon this basic educational foundation as they began to develop their clinical skills. Although at a baccalaureate level these potential counselors were not advanced statisticians, they did understand empirical method well enough to understand what a piece of research was attempting to demonstrate. They also were able to understand, in general, what the result of a diagnostic test was revealing to them.

One other observation that I was able to make was that whether or not a potential counselor was in recovery from addictions had absolutely no bearing on whether or not he or she could be effective as a chemical dependency counselor. The determining factor in making a distinction between who became an effective counselor and who did not was, more than anything, education.

Again, I would have to pose the question: is it reasonable to assume that persons who are given what is presumed to be the equivalent of six to seven college classes in terms of education, and then offered six thousand hours of supervised experience exposing them to only one singular method of treating a disorder, should be considered to be qualified to provide treatment for any disorder? I don't see how we can make such an assumption. If such an assumption was made with regard to the treatment of any other mental disorder, it would be violating ethical standards and moral obligations. Moreover, to do so would be illegal in any state within this nation.

What is even more incredulous is that in some states, a person might complete a master's degree in psychology, counseling, or social work, complete all other requirements to become licensed as a mental health professional, and still not be allowed to provide treatment for addictions. I have seen this happen many times. A counselor with a master's degree and professional credentials will frequently have to spend at least one year, or two thousand hours, under the supervision of a licensed or certified chemical dependency counselor to become eligible for licensure or certification as a chemical dependency counselor. When this happens, it is not at all unusual to see a master's level counselor under the supervision of a chemical dependency counselor who has never even attended college.

Some state authorities have made attempts to justify such practices by stating that the person's degree program did not specifically offer training in the understanding and treatment of addictions. Personally, I have always found this excuse to be ridiculous.

Alcohol and drug abuse is specifically addressed in any abnormal psychology class offered either as an undergraduate class or as a graduate-level class in counseling programs on every college campus that offers accredited counseling training. It is also addressed in other college course offerings as well. I have come to believe that the justification used by state authorities in their insistence that a master's level counselor should be supervised by a less-qualified individual really means that the counselor training program did not offer adequate indoctrination into twelve-step ideology!

There are even more problems that become obvious when an attempt is made to justify the practices employed in twelve-step treatment in comparison to ethical standards that serve as a guide to the variety of the helping professions. For example, the ethical standards pertaining to the counseling profession and twelve-step treatment are, in many instances, obviously incompatible. This becomes very problematic when one considers that most professional codes of ethics are directly related to state and federal laws that regulate standards of professional practice and provide guidelines for the protection of patients' rights. No matter what professional code of ethics one would wish to examine (that of medicine, psychology, professional counseling, drug and alcohol counseling, etc.), there are certain core principles that guide the legal and ethical practice of these disciplines. Ethical and moral concepts that are common in all of the helping professions include beneficence, non-malfeasance (doing no harm), individual autonomy, and justice.

Also common to all ethical codes, and to the legal codes in all fifty states governing the practice of medical and mental health treatment, is the legal standard of informed consent. The ethical concepts listed above are all related in some way to legal standards of informed consent. The right to informed consent is afforded to all competent adults. Parents or legal guardians must provide informed consent for children to be offered treatment of any kind. To commence with the provision of any form of treatment, the individual practitioners or the treatment organization must secure informed consent from a prospective patient, unless the circumstances constitute a life-threatening emergency or the individual patient is determined to be incompetent to provide their consent.

The American Medical Association (2005) offers the following description of what is considered to be sufficient in terms of affording informed consent to a prospective patient:

> In the communication process, the physician providing or performing the treatment and/or procedure (not a delegated representative) should disclose and discuss with the patient: the patient's diagnosis, if known; the nature and the purpose of a proposed treatment or procedure; the risks and benefits of a proposed treatment or procedure; alternatives (regardless of their cost or the extent to which the treatment options are covered by health insurance); the risks and benefits of the alternative treatment or procedure; and the risks and benefits of not receiving or undergoing a treatment or procedure.

In turn, the patient should have the opportunity to ask questions to elicit a better understanding of the treatment or procedure, so that he or she can make an informed decision to proceed or to refuse a particular course of medical intervention. Informed consent, as described, is legally required in all fifty states and for all forms of treatment, whether that treatment is for a medical problem, a mental problem, or an alcohol- or drug-related problem. This right of informed consent is based on the common belief that individuals have the right to control access to their own bodies (which includes the mind) and to make informed decisions about their own health and well-being (decisions with which others might disagree), and live or die with the consequences (Canterbury v. Spence, 1972; Natanson v. Kline, 1960). Courts have repeatedly affirmed that a person has a right to refuse (even one who is hospitalized for mental illness, if competent) any and all medical treatment (e.g., Rogers v. Commissioner of the Department of Mental Health, 1983).

In the addictions treatment industry, informed consent is frequently ignored completely, or at the very least significantly sidestepped. Many thousands of people are routinely mandated into addictions treatment by courts or coerced by private employers during the course of any given year (Peele and Brodsky, 1991; Wiesner, 1990). The vast majority of these individuals are offered no choices in the treatment to which they must submit. These coerced individuals are not informed about alternative treatments that have had better outcome records in clinical research (Miller et al., 1995). Issues of outpatient versus inpatient treatment are similarly decided based on what a given program might offer (and what the patients' insurance might cover) rather than proven efficacy (Miller and Hester, 1986).

When you consider that most of the addiction counselors that work in treatment programs across the nation know little or nothing about anything other than twelve-step treatment, could it reasonably be expected that they would be able to discuss alternative treatments with their patients in order to provide the patient with sufficient information to get informed consent? Considering the limited ability that many of these addiction counselors have to accurately interpret the results of scientific literature, could they even provide their clients with accurate information regarding the relative efficacy of any variety of treatment approaches? Considering these addictions counselors' devotion to AA doctrine, could they or would they be able to accurately discuss the potential risks to the patient relative to any choices that might be made by the client regarding their treatment? Could they even be counted on to provide their patients with a reliable and valid diagnosis of their problems? This comprises just some of the questions that arise when one examines the qualifications of many addictions counselors in an effort to access their ability to function as true professionals in a treatment setting.

> Do practitioners in the addictions treatment industry really ignore, or sidestep, the rights of their patients in this way? The answer to this question is undeniably yes. It happens frequently and regularly.

One practice particularly common among counselors who adhere to AA doctrine is that which is frequently referred to as intervention. This is a practice which is completely inconsistent with the standard of informed consent. In the intervention, an individual is surrounded by his or her friends, family, and very often a treatment professional. Collectively, the family members, friends, and the counselor confront the individual in an attempt to convince the patient that he or she has become out of control and the individual needs treatment for addiction. This process very closely resembles what was described in a previous chapter as being "the hot seat" employed within treatment group sessions (see Chapter Five).

If all goes as planned, the individual who has been the target of the intervention is immediately whisked off to a treatment center whereat the individual's admittance had been prearranged, most often by the counselor who led the intervention.

I have been a party to two of these interventions. My participation in the interventions was as a family member in one instance and a friend of the targeted individual in the other instance. I can assure the reader that such interventions are extremely intensive and coercive in nature. In essence, with the guidance of the so-called treatment professional, friends and family verbally badger and brutalize the targeted individual until he or she either submits to the desires of the group, or simply leaves the site where the intervention is commencing. In one of these instances, the confrontation even became physical at times. This process called intervention cannot be described as being anything other than coercion. Although, I have heard some counselors state that such interventions are done in the name of "tough love."

My participation in these both of theses interventions occurred prior to my entering into professional training. Once I had been exposed to the concepts of professional ethics, it became clear to me that I would never participate in such an intervention in any capacity.

Additionally, my conceptualization of "tough love" is that you allow an individual to make his or her own decisions regarding life, while recognizing that he or she must also be accountable for whatever might become of the individual's decisions. It doesn't involve coercing anyone into doing what you, or someone else, might consider to be best for the individual. Again, in what world can such practices be justified as being done in the name of treatment? Only in the world that subscribes to AA doctrine!

In times that have thankfully passed, major treatment providers would actually employ addictions counselors, and others, to go out into the community specifically to conduct interventions and thereby recruit patients into their alcohol and drug treatment programs. Individuals that were employed in this capacity were referred to as "headhunters," and they were paid a "bounty" for every individual that they referred, or coerced, into treatment. Frequently, these headhunters would align themselves with schools, probation officers, medical professionals, law enforcement, and even courts to search out situations wherein they could offer their services to intervene into a family or other set of circumstances to coerce an individual into treatment. This was a relatively routine practice up until about fifteen years ago. Most states have since taken steps to legally prohibit such practices today.

In his book *Bedlam: Greed, Profiteering, and Fraud in a Mental Health System Gone Crazy* (1994), author J. Sharkey described how treatment providers in Texas actually employed security guards to round up suspected substance abusers. The victims of this practice would assume that they were being placed under arrest by law enforcement. Once they were "arrested" they were taken and deposited in for-profit hospitals. Eventually, State Senator Frank Tejeda introduced legislation that caused Texas to crack down on such illegal and unethical practices.

As can be seen, the legal requirement of informed consent has not always been given high priority in the addictions treatment industry. Historically, it had been largely ignored by twelve-step treatment providers. This is evidenced going clear back to the early days in Akron, Ohio, where Dr. Bob first began to provide twelve-step treatment. As was indicated in the previous chapter, "The alcoholic himself didn't ask for help. He didn't have anything to say about it" (Alcoholics Anonymous, 1980). In many respects it hasn't changed that much to the present day. Rigid adherence to twelve-step ideology to the exclusion of all other conceivable treatment alternatives practically ensures that individuals entering into over 90 percent of the treatment programs in this nation will not be afforded the right of informed consent. Can you envision that a treatment provider would actually sit and accurately describe the treatment as follows?

1. We have diagnosed you as suffering from a substance use mental disorder. We are convinced, according to AA doctrine, that you actually suffer from a disease, which we cannot verify by any scientific means.

2. We are recommending that you would benefit most by being treated according to the Minnesota Model, which is intensive exposure to the first four steps of AA, followed by lifelong membership in a twelve-step support group.

3. There are alternatives to the treatment we are recommending that have been scientifically proven to be more effective than what we are recommending. In fact, the treatment we recommend may not be even as effective as no treatment at all. But, we believe it is the only way to treat this disease because this is all we know how to do.

4. The risk for you, should you decide to participate in this treatment, is that it will be extremely expensive, and it may not work for you.

5. The risk for you, should you decide not to partake of the treatment we recommend, is that you will either get worse, or you might actually experience spontaneous recovery without treatment. Or, another treatment method might be more effective for you, but we don't actually know what these methods are.

6. We will respect your decision, no matter what that might be.

Would this really happen? I don't think so! In essence, in the treatment industry even as it exists today, informed consent really doesn't mean much.

Is the neglect of legal and ethical standards within the addictions treatment industry limited to the principle of informed consent? We will examine some other ethical principles that are codified in relation to the practices of alcohol and drug counselors to see if other standards, ethical or legal, might be ignored.

Many states have established codes of ethics for chemical dependency counselors who are either identical, or very similar, to those utilized by NAADAC. Since this is the case, we will examine the ethical standards that NAADAC (2005) has established for those counselors who are certified by that organization.

NAADAC Principle 1. Non-discrimination.

The NAADAC member shall not discriminate against client or professionals based on race, *religion*, age, gender, disability, national ancestry, sexual orientation, or economic condition [emphasis added].

As you can see, I have emphasized the word religion as it is stated within this first ethical principle. It was previously mentioned that many thousands of individuals are coerced into twelve-step treatment programs by their employers, professional organizations, or they are mandated by the courts to attend treatment. Since most counselors that are certified by NAADAC strongly adhere to twelve-step ideology, and the entirety of the Twelve Steps makes constant reference to God, it seems very likely that many who are guided by this ethical standard violate it on a frequent and regular basis.

The references made to God in the Twelve Steps have been a source of much controversy over many years. AA and its promoters have consistently asserted that the word God used in the Twelve Steps does not necessarily mean that a person must submit to Christian beliefs to find recovery in their programs. Regardless of this assertion, several important court decisions, including *Arnold v. Tennessee Board of Paroles* (1997), *Warner V. Orange County Department of Probation* (2nd Cir., 1997), *Griffin V. Coughlin* (New York, 1996), *Rauser V. Horn* (3rd Cir., 2001), and *Kerr V. Farrey* (7th Cir., 1996) have defined

Alcoholics Anonymous and other treatment programs based on AA's Twelve Steps as being religious in nature (Peele, 2001).

Essentially, in these cases the courts found that compelling individuals to participate in AA or in twelve-step treatment did constitute a violation of the First Amendment's separation-of-church-and-state clause. Despite these rulings, twelve-step programs continue to require that patients required to attend treatment by their employers, professional organizations, and even the courts adhere to twelve-step doctrine. Additionally, as was evidenced in previous chapters, treatment activities in many treatment programs may require individuals to participate in the Lord's Prayer and the Serenity Prayer. The former can be found in any Christian bible.

Personally, I subscribe to Christian beliefs in my own life. Professionally, I recognize that any attempt on my part to force my religious beliefs onto a patient, or even an individual who is not a patient, would constitute a violation of my professional ethics as well as being a violation of individual's legal rights.

We can now see that, at least in some instances, addictions counselors who are employed within twelve-step treatment programs, or even some in private practice, are likely to be in violation of their ethical principles when they require their patients to adhere to twelve-step treatment.

NAADAC Principle 2. Responsibility.

b. The NAADAC member, as educator, has a primary obligation to help others acquire knowledge and skills in dealing with the *disease of alcoholism and drug abuse* [emphasis added].

Since it has been clearly demonstrated that the disease concept of alcoholism or addiction to other substances cannot be supported by any scientific means, how can NAADAC assume that it is ethical to perpetuate this myth? Is it ethical to attempt to convince patients, or the general public, to accept as fact something that is clearly not a fact?

While I would concede that most people in the addictions treatment industry adhere to this mistaken concept, the mere fact that most people might believe something to be true does not mean that it is the truth. This certainly demonstrates how strongly NAADAC supports AA ideology. Unfortunately, since most states have adopted codes of ethics that state exactly what is stated in NAADAC's principle, it would appear that AA doctrine also is equally predominant within the licensing authorities of these states as well.

> **c. The NAADAC member who supervises others accepts the obligation to facilitate further professional development of these individuals by providing *accurate and current information*, timely evaluations, and constructive consultation [emphasis added].**

If NAADAC supervisors support and follow this principle, why is it that so many addictions counselors, especially those certified by NAADAC, know nothing about other treatment approaches? If NAADAC supervisors can understand the scientific literature currently existing within the treatment field, why do many of them continue to promote twelve-step treatment exclusively?

> *NAADAC Principle 4: Legal and Moral Standards.*
>
> **a. The NAADAC member shall be fully cognizant of all federal laws and laws of the member's respective state governing the practice of alcoholism and drug abuse counseling.**

We have already examined the legal requirement of informed consent. We have also examined First Amendment violations. Addictions counselors, either those certified by NAADAC or their respective state authorities, who continue to work in twelve-step treatment programs that accept mandated patients into treatment and who continue to require those patients to adhere to twelve-step treatment, are violating the legal rights of those who have come to them for help. Their behavior cannot be considered to be ethical in light of these legal violations.

I could go on and examine the remaining ethical principles that comprise the ethical standards adopted by NAADAC and many of the various states that have adopted similar ethical standards. I believe that what is outlined herein more than proves my point. Simply stated, rigid adherence to twelve-step doctrine in the provision of treatment to individuals who suffer from substance use disorders can no longer be considered to be an ethical practice. In many instances, individuals who are offered such treatment and are not informed about or given access to other forms of treatment have been subjected to violations of both ethical and legal standards. Their rights have been violated and they have been subjected to costly treatment that has proven to be the least effective form of treatment available.

In this chapter we have covered much ground. We have examined treatment based on the Minnesota Model, or twelve-step approach, and its ability to provide individuals with treatment based on the individual's specific needs. We have discovered that such treatment cannot meet this requirement. As such, the "one approach cures all ills" treatment cannot meet the licensing standards relative to the provision of individualized treatment.

We have examined the qualifications of certified and/or licensed chemical dependency counselors. What we find, in many instances, is that these treatment providers cannot be considered to be qualified relative to the same standards that we would expect of professionals offering treatment for any other mental disorder. We can certainly find cause to question if many of these so-called counselors are actually qualified to treat anything at all.

We have examined twelve-step treatment in relation to its ability to conform to legal and ethical standards. We have discovered that, by its very nature, twelve-step treatment is incapable of meeting some ethical or legal standards. As such, counselors who rigidly adhere to twelve-step doctrine may frequently and regularly violate both the legal and ethical standards that govern their profession.

Misfeasance refers to the "improper and unlawful execution of an act that in itself is lawful and proper" (*Webster's II New Riverside*

Dictionary, 1984). Certainly it is lawful and proper to offer a proven remedy to an individual who suffers from a mental disorder. On the other hand, is it really lawful and proper to allow the remedy to be rendered by those who are ill-qualified to do so? Is it lawful and proper to provide the remedy in ways that, with respect to any other mental illness, would be considered unethical and illegal? I believe that twelve-step treatment along with those who rigidly adhere to and continue to promote twelve-step doctrine have been weighed and measured. By any reasonable and logical standard, proponents of this approach have been found to be legally, ethically, and morally wanting!

References

Chapter Six

Alcoholics Anonymous. (1980). *Dr. Bob and the Good Oldtimers.* (pp. 82–83). New York, NY: Alcoholics Anonymous World Services, Inc.

American Medical Association. (2005). Informed consent. Web site: http://www.ama-assn.org/ama/pub/category/4608.html.

Anderson, D. J., McGovern, J. P., and DuPont, R. L. (1999). The origins of the Minnesota model of addiction—A first person account. American Society of Addiction Medicine. *Journal of Addictive Disease,* **18(4).**

Bufe, C. (1998). AA's impact on society. *Alcoholics Anonymous: Cult or Cure.* 2nd edition, revised. San Francisco, CA: See Sharp Press.

Canterbury v. Spence. (1972). 464 F2d 772 (DC Cir.), cert. den., 409 U.S. 1064.

Miller, W. R., and Hester, R. K. (1986). Inpatient alcoholism treatment: Who benefits? *American Psychologist,* **41,** 794–805.

Miller, W. R., Brown, J. M., Simpson, T. L., Handmaker, N. S., Bien, T. H., Luckie, L. F., Montgomery, H. A., et al. (1995). What works? A methodological analysis of the alcohol treatment outcome literature. R. K. Hester and W. R. Miller (eds.), *Handbook of alcoholism treatment approaches* (2nd ed., pp. 12–44). Boston, MA: Allyn and Bacon.

Natanson v. Kline. (1960). 186 Kan 393, 350 P2d 1093.

National Association of Alcohol and Drug Abuse Counselors. (2005). Eligibility requirements for national certified addiction counselor credential, level 1. Web site: http://www.naadac.org.

National Association of Alcohol and Drug Abuse Counselors. (2005). Ethical standards for counselors by the NAADAC, The Association for Addictions Professionals. Web site: http://www. naadac.org.

Peele, S. (2001). Is AA's loss psychology's gain? *Monitor on Psychology*, **35(7)**, 86.

Peele, S., and Brodsky, A. (1991). What's up to doc? *Reason*, 34–36.

Rogers v. Commissioner of the Department of Mental Health. (1983). 390 Mass. 489, 458 NE2d 308.

Sharkey, J. (1994). *Bedlam: Greed, Profiteering, and Fraud in a Mental Health System Gone Crazy.* New York, NY: St. Martin's Press.

State of Nebraska. (1998). *Title 20: Regulations for Certifying Alcohol/ Drug Abuse Counselors under the Division of Alcoholism, Drug Abuse and Addictions Services.* Department of Health and Human Services. Division of Alcoholism, Drug Abuse and Addictions Services, Lincoln, Nebraska.

University of Nebraska at Kearney. (1999). *2004–2006 Undergraduate Catalog.* Kearney, Nebraska. Web site: http://www.unk.edu/ acad.

Webster's II New Riverside Dictionary (1984). Boston, MA: A Berkley Book published by Houghton Mifflin, p. 450.

Weisner, C. M. (1990). Coercion in alcohol treatment. *Broadening the Base of Treatment for Alcohol Problems.* Institute of Medicine,

Division of Mental Health and Behavioral Medicine. (pp. 579–609). Washington, DC: National Academy Press.

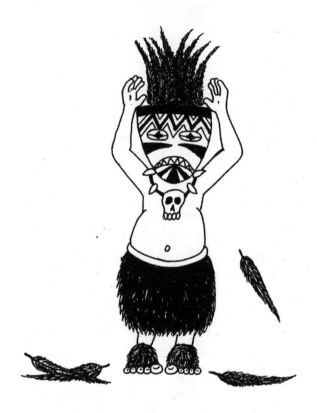

Chapter Seven

Misconceptualization: Failure to Operationally Define Addiction

We know that addiction to alcohol and other mood-altering substances cannot be considered a disease. Yet, it is rather apparent the addictions treatment industry has actively promoted this disease concept from the days of its early development to the present day. Since the emergence of Alcoholics Anonymous in the 1930s to this day, the notion that alcoholics and addicts are somehow mentally and physically distinct from other individuals has been perpetuated by AA and those who actively promote AA doctrine. As such, the belief that individuals who suffer from alcoholism and other addictions should appropriately be treated in a manner that is completely divorced from the treatment of all other mental disorders, or any other physical illness, has also been perpetuated. The result of this continual and vehement promotion of the disease concept of addiction, in accordance to AA doctrine, is that we now find that our nation, state by state, is heavily invested in the creation, maintenance, and perpetuation of a form of treatment which has proven to be no more effective than providing no treatment at all. It even appears that many efforts devoted to the treatment of addictions are unethical in their practices and, in some instances, actually violate the legal rights of the individuals that these efforts are attempting to treat.

Something has to change. To complacently sit back and allow things to remain as they are is simply not an option. If we, collectively, fail to take corrective action in our efforts to combat addictions, many millions of our nation's citizens will continue to suffer needlessly.

Considering the massive drain on our nation's resources posed by the ever-expanding problem of substance abuse, it may well be that the very survival of our nation may depend, at least to some extent, on our ability to come to grips with these problems.

Change is never easy. This is particularly true when change requires that we must abandon beliefs and practices held to be true for very long periods of time. For example, how long did it take man to accept the notion that the earth was not the center of the universe? Or, that the earth was round as opposed to the notion that it was flat? When you can fully appreciate the kind of changes required of us to alter the course of addiction treatment within our nation, it stands to reason that opposition to those changes will be extremely dramatic and enduring. Nonetheless, changes must be made.

Where do we start? Earlier, I recalled a comment that had been offered by one my former college professors. The comment offered was to the effect of, "If you can't accurately diagnose the patient's problem, how can you ever expect to devise a way to effectively treat his or her problem?" The professor's words have been constantly reinforced in my work with patients over the years. Whatever success I can claim regarding my efforts to help patients overcome their problems has always been dependent on my ability to accurately conceptualize what they were experiencing. In other words, if I could accurately diagnose and define what my patient was actually experiencing, I consistently found that I was able to devise treatments which resulted in better outcomes.

It should be very clear by now that I have always seen the reliance on the disease concept of addiction to be a major stumbling block in developing an ability to effectively treat addiction. Simply stated, it is a gross misconceptualization! The fact that treatment efforts that have relied on the disease concept have proven to be wholly ineffective should serve as ample support to this basic assertion. More than 90 percent of the treatment programs in this nation have prescribed a spiritual or mystical method of treating what they have commonly believed to be a "primary, chronic disease with genetic, psychosocial, and environmental factors influencing its development and manifestations" (NCADD, 2005). This clearly indicates how horribly mistaken and misguided such efforts have been.

The mistakes begin with the assumption that addiction is a disease. What is it that distinguishes the alcoholic or the addict from you, me, the next-door neighbor lady, the local butcher, the banker, the grocer, or your local clergyman? The common belief has been that the addict is "bodily and mentally different" (Alcoholics Anonymous, 1939) from other individuals. However, as we have already demonstrated, there is no medical or other scientific evidence that suggests that the alcoholic or addict is in any way bodily or mentally different from anybody else. The only way that we can distinguish the alcoholic or the addict from any other human being is by his or her behavior!

Behavior is the standard by which the mental disorder of substance dependence is defined. *The Diagnostic and Statistical Manual of Mental Disorders, Fourth Edition* (DSM-IV) (American Psychiatric Association, 1994) defines substance dependence as follows:

> A maladaptive pattern of substance use, leading to clinically significant impairment or distress, as manifested by three or more of the following, occurring at any time in the same 12-month period:

1. tolerance, as defined by either of the following:
   a. a need for markedly increased amounts of the substance to achieve intoxication or desired effect
   b. markedly diminished effect with continued use of the same amount of the substance
2. withdrawal, as manifested by either of the following:
   a. the characteristic withdrawal syndrome for the substance
   b. the same substance (or a closely related) substance is taken to relieve or avoid withdrawal symptoms
3. the substance is often taken in larger amounts over a longer period than was intended
4. there is a persistent desire or unsuccessful efforts to cut down or control substance use

5. a great deal of time is spent in activities necessary to obtain the substance (e.g. visiting multiple doctors or driving long distances), use the substance, or recover from its effects
6. important social, occupational, or recreational activities are given up or reduced because of substance use
7. the substance use is continued despite knowledge of having a persistent or recurring physical or psychological problem that is likely to have been caused or exacerbated by the substance. (p. 181)

It can be specified if the patient can be seen as being physiologically dependent on the substance, and course specifiers can be listed as well.

As can be seen, the DSM-IV qualifies a diagnosis of substance dependence in strictly behavioral terms. There is no mention of any physiological criteria that has been established as a means to identify a person who is presumed to be dependent upon a given substance save that of tolerance and withdrawal. Even then, these are defined in terms of observable behavior. The DSM-IV does not define substance dependence as a disease.

The DSM-IV provides us with the accepted systematic procedures for arriving at a reliable and valid diagnosis for all recognized mental disorders. Substance dependence, or addiction, is regarded as being among all the recognized mental disorders, not separate from them. Comparing an individual's behavior according to these accepted behavioral criteria is how professionals that work within all the helping professions systematically arrive at a reliable and valid diagnosis of substance dependence.

Many professionals that work within the addictions treatment industry do utilize the DSM-IV in some manner. In fact, many states require that programs licensed for addiction treatment list patients' diagnoses according to the terminology provided by the DSM-IV. All third-party payers (e.g., private insurance, Medicare, Medicaid, etc.) require that diagnoses should be made according to DSM-IV criteria. With that said, I will reiterate that I have met many licensed or certified chemical dependency counselors that have never even seen a full-text version of this manual. Many addictions counselors do not know how to fully utilize this tool.

The primary utility of the DSM-IV is that of a diagnostic aide. It is, however, a very advanced and complex tool that holds a great deal of valuable information about various mental disorders that can be used in research, treatment planning, and other clinical activities. To fully understand the many uses that can be made of this valuable tool requires that the user has a relatively advanced knowledge of abnormal behavior, statistics and empirical inquiry, medical terminology, sociology, and other disciplines. Simply stated, there are many addictions counselors who lack the educational background that is needed to utilize this tool to its full potential.

The DSM-IV provides mental health professionals with a means of identifying specific mental disorders. It does not really attempt to convey a complete conceptualization of any mental disorder. The DSM-IV does not specifically convey what causes mental disorders nor does it offer recommendations as to how treat the various mental disorders.

Being able to accurately identify substance dependence according to behavioral criteria is just one facet of deriving an operational conceptualization of this disorder, albeit an important one. I choose to use the term "operational conceptualization" because that conveys that the clinician is not merely attempting to simply identify what disorder his or her patient might be suffering, but he or she is also attempting to create a workable overall mental image of what substance dependence might mean for the individual patient who is seeking treatment. In that context, rendering a construct to be operational means, as much as possible, to take something that is intangible, such as a mental disorder, and make it usable by defining it in concrete terms. This is why mental disorders are most often defined in terms of the observable behaviors most frequently associated with a specific disorder. Behavior is observable and can be measured in relatively concrete terms.

To form a complete and useful operational conceptualization of addiction, it is important to be able to understand, as much as possible, all the various factors which contribute to the development of addiction. By factors, I mean all those characteristics that might exist within an individual, combined with all the influences originating from the individual's environment, and how the interactions between the individual and the environment might combine to create a condition wherein the individual engages in the compulsive use of a mood-altering substance.

This sounds very complicated, doesn't it? Would you really want to assign this task to someone whose whole understanding of human behavior is based on the equivalent of six or seven college classes? Understanding abnormal behavior is complicated. That's why individuals who generally work in professional fields that attempt to treat mental disorders such as psychologists, psychiatrists, professional counselors, and so on, are required to invest many years in gaining the educational foundations and the experiential guidance that is required to prepare them to take on such complicated tasks!

Developing an "operational conceptualization" is an important initial component of any approach to the treatment of mental disorders. It allows the clinician to view the patient's problem from more of a holistic perspective. It allows the clinician to be able to consider all the various factors that have contributed to the development of a given mental disorder. This, in turn, enables the clinician to devise strategies that might positively impact the patient's problems by specifically targeting the factors that are likely to have caused the problem the patient is now presenting. In other words, creating an operational conceptualization of the patient's problem enables the clinician to devise a treatment plan that is target-specific.

As was inferred in the previous chapter, the concept of target specificity in planning the treatment of addicted persons has been all but completely absent within the addictions treatment industry as it has evolved, and as it currently exists. The stubborn reliance on the disease concept of addiction characteristic of all twelve-step treatment programs is prohibitive of target specificity primarily because the disease concept, at its very roots, assumes that addiction is a phenomenon that is pretty much the same for all individuals. In other words, all addicts suffer from the same disease; therefore, addiction is the same for everyone.

All twelve-step treatment programs apply exactly the same core treatment for every person. The individual completes the first four of the Twelve Steps in a treatment environment, followed by an effort directed toward convincing the person that they must continue to work the Twelve Steps by committing themselves to prolonged, sometimes lifelong, membership in a Twelve Step support group such as AA.

This lack of consideration for the individual patient's experience of addiction is made even worse by the fact that all too often the addictions counselors who guide the treatment of the addicted person are, themselves, recovering from a substance-dependence disorder. So, in addition to applying a "one method cures all" approach to treating the addicted person, the recovering counselor will frequently assume that his or her patient must follow the same "path to recovery" that the counselor experienced in recovery. Frequently, if the recovering addictions counselor perceives that the patient is not conducting his or her recovery effort according to the counselor's perception of what constitutes an adequate or proper effort, the patient is terminated from treatment because the counselor considers the patient to be noncompliant.

It is very evident that twelve-step treatment is a very errant and restrictive form of treatment. First, it assumes that addiction is the same "disease" for all addicted persons. Second, it assumes that all addicted persons can be effectively treated by applying the exact same treatment method. Then, it is not at all unusual for the treatment to be made even more narrow and restrictive in accordance with the recovering counselor's perceptions that he or she acquired as a result of his or her own personal recovery.

Each patient's experience of any given mental disorder is unique to that patient. For example, depression is not the same for all individuals who experience depressive symptoms. Anxiety problems are different from individual to individual. Compulsions are different from one individual to another, and so on. Substance dependence is no exception.

As the experiences that come from suffering from any given mental problem differ from individual to individual, so do the causes of these problems. The specific factors that contribute to the depression experienced by one individual are always slightly different from those which cause another individual to become depressed. Similarly, the various factors that might combine to cause one individual to abuse mood-altering substances may be completely different from those which cause another individual to engage in the compulsive use of mood-altering substances. Simply stated, substance use disorders are not the same phenomenon for every individual. Different factors within the individual, from within the individual's environment and in the interactions of the two, combine to contribute to the development of substance use problems that are unique to each person. Addiction cannot be viewed as being the same problem for everyone that experiences addiction. As such, no singular approach to treating addictions, such as the Twelve Steps, can be expected to be effective for all people who suffer from addictions.

Assuming that there is only one way to treat addiction is absurd. We cannot assume that we can treat all depression by applying one specific treatment to all who suffer from depression. We cannot expect to be able to treat any given mental problem by applying one singular treatment method to all who might suffer from that mental problem. Yet, the addictions treatment industry, as it has evolved to its current form, stubbornly insists all addictions can be treated through the application of a single treatment approach. It is really no surprise that these efforts have, historically, been unable to demonstrate positive results.

Treatment for any problem must be designed according to what the individual patient is experiencing, and upon the various factors that might be identified as contributors to the problem. Effective treatment does not depend entirely upon the clinician's perceptions, expectations, desires, or beliefs. Effective treatment can only be devised if it is designed according to the individual patient's needs!

Effective treatment begins when the clinician acquires an operational conceptualization of what "substance dependence" means to the individual patient. That is, the clinician must be able to identify the disorder, understand what factors within the individual might contribute to the problem, and understand how the influences coming from the individual's environment might have contributed to the observed disorder. If the clinician can accomplish this conceptualization, even to a modest degree, he or she stands a much better chance of devising a plan to treat the individual that will specifically target those factors that caused the patient to become dependent upon mood-altering substances.

What are the factors that cause addiction? I wish that this question could be answered simply by listing some common causes for these problems. The truth is substance dependence is a very complex problem. The factors that combine to cause individuals to engage in the compulsive use of mood-altering substances frequently vary a great deal from person to person. As variable as the factors that contribute to the development of substance use disorders appear to be when making comparisons between individuals, there are also some factors that appear repeatedly among substance-dependent persons as a group. We will attempt to examine some of those factors which contribute heavily to the development of substance use disorders.

First, we need to examine which factors within individuals seem to be, generally, characteristic of substance abusers.

We have already looked at genetics as a cause for addiction. There is absolutely no evidence suggesting that we can identify a potential addict in terms of his or her genetics. The current body of research conducted up to this point in time merely suggests that there may be any number of genes or gene combinations that may render a given person vulnerable in some way to certain chemicals. Findings from such research certainly have not led us to a point wherein we can generalize how genetics might contribute to addiction. Since no human being can be considered an example of genetic perfection, as if such a thing could even be recognized, we all have genetic vulnerabilities to something.

We have looked at neurotransmission as a potential contributor to addiction. Current research has yielded no evidence demonstrating the existence of readily identifiable abnormalities in human neurotransmission processes that can be isolated as contributing factors in the development of addictions.

To date, there is no valid scientific evidence of a physiological cause for addiction! That does not mean that the physical health of a substance-dependent patient is not a concern. We all know that the repeated and prolonged use of alcohol and other drugs causes physical damage to the substance-dependent person. We also know that the introduction of mood-altering substances into the human body is very likely to cause the patient's brain to function in ways that can be considered to be abnormal, to varying degrees, depending upon the substance used and the extent of the patient's use. As this is often the case, substance-dependent patients should always be required to undergo thorough medical examinations. If it is determined that a patient is in need of medical treatment, the patient should certainly be encouraged to accept such treatment.

There has been a considerable amount of research which has looked to the possibility that individuals might be vulnerable to addiction because they possess certain psychological characteristics. We will look at a few examples of such inquiry.

The possibility that individuals who fall victim to addictions may suffer from defects in character, or abnormal personality traits, has been a matter of debate even prior to the publication of Freud's theories. Some have gone so far as to attempt to describe what has been referred to as an "addictive personality" (Miessner, 1980). Generally speaking, descriptions of what might have been considered characteristic traits of this personality type have been vague and inconsistent. The consensus at the present time is that little evidence points to the existence of a specific personality that might be prone toward addiction (Dodes, 2002; Lugwig, 1988).

Most professionals in the addiction fields have rejected the notion that addicts come from a specific personality type. Yet, there is evidence suggesting that substance abusers, as a whole, do exhibit some similar characteristics, or personality traits. The Minnesota Muiltiphasic Personality Inventory (MMPI) is a personality assessment instrument that has gained wide acceptance in its use in many clinical and research settings (Hathaway and McKinley, 1943). The MMPI consists of a number of empirically validated scales that assess various facets of personality. Two MMPI scales have consistently been utilized as one means of identifying alcoholics with a relatively high degree of reliability.

The first MMPI scale that appeared to be able to identify alcoholics is the PD or Psycho Deviate scale. High scorers on this scale have frequently been found to have a potential for the development of alcoholism. This scale gauges the individual's disregard for social customs and mores, his or her relative ability to benefit from punishing experiences, the individual's emotional shallowness, and the individual's inability to create intimate relationships. Zucker and Gomberg (1986) summarized a range of studies which indicated that boys who subsequently become alcoholics were characterized by their superficial relationships throughout life.

The second of these scales is the MAC scale which was developed by Craig MacAndrew. MacAndrew (1981) asserted that individuals who achieve high scores on this scale have an "assertive, aggressive, pleasure-seeking character" which made those who appear to be alcoholics to "resemble criminals and delinquents" (p. 617). It has been stated that 75 to 85 percent of all patients could be correctly placed in the psychiatric or alcoholic category by relying on the patient's MAC score. The scale appears to work equally well in identifying both men and woman (MacAndrew, 1986a).

MacAndrew found that adolescent drinkers who had been treated for alcohol problems also achieved elevated MAC scores. He modified the MAC scale for this younger group to create a new scale, the Substance Abuse Proclivity scale (SAP), which has demonstrated to be a reliable predictor of problem drinking and drug abuse in youth ages sixteen to twenty-five years (MacAndrew, 1986b).

The ability of the SAP scale to identify young substance abusers offers a reasonable argument that there may be certain personality traits that might be predictive of an individual's potential for becoming a substance abuser. This hypothesis has been tested by several research efforts which supported this notion. Hoffman et al. (1974) and Loper et al. (1973) compared MMPI scores of college students who later became alcoholics with those who did not. The MMPI scores between the two groups showed differences very similar to those that noted according to the MAC scale, indicating that those whose scored higher levels of sociopathy, defiance of authority, and impulsiveness, were more likely to later become alcoholics

What we see as a result of these efforts is that individuals who exhibit personality traits, including sociopathy, assertiveness, aggressiveness, pleasure-seeking, defiance of authority, impulsivity, and the inability to form stable and lasting relationships, may have a propensity to abuse alcohol and other substances. These characteristics, or traits, appear to be related to addiction according to how they are defined and measured by the MMPI.

While it may be very important to understand that addicts may present with some common personality traits or characteristics, it must also be made very clear that the traits listed above can be associated with a number of different personality types. For example, aggressiveness, impulsivity, and an inability to form stable relationships are listed as characteristics that can be observed, to varying degrees, in individuals that might present with any personality disorder described in the DSM-IV (pp. 629–673).

Anyone who has spent significant time treating addicted persons can attest to the fact that the personalities or characterological styles of the individuals they have treated vary significantly. I have observed no single personality type that can be consistently associated with addiction. Addiction to mood-altering substances appears to occur across the entire spectrum of the possible characterological styles that one might observe in others in clinical practice, or even in day-to-day life. However, individuals who do become dependent upon mood-altering substances frequently exhibit varying combinations of those characteristics identified by MMPI (sociopathy, assertiveness, aggressiveness, impulsiveness, pleasure-seeking, defiance of authority, an inability to form stable and lasting relationships, etc.). A thorough clinical history of these individuals frequently indicates that expressions of these characteristics were exhibited by these individuals prior to the onset of substance use.

Confusing, isn't it? Let us define some terms to clarify some of this confusion.

Personality is defined as the "organization of relatively enduring characteristics unique to an individual, as revealed by the individual's interaction with his or her environment" (Dworetzky, 1982).

A personality disorder is defined as "deeply ingrained, habitual, and rigid patterns of behavior or character that severely limit the adaptive potential of the individual but that are often not seen by him or her to be problematic or maladaptive. Sometimes called character disorders" (Ibid).

As can be seen, an individual's personality consists of a number of various characteristics or traits, that combine in such a way as to guide how he or she might interact with the environment. A personality disorder exists when these characteristics develop in such a way as to become rigid, habitual, and maladaptive to such an extent that the individual cannot function within or interact normally with his or her environment.

Generally speaking, past efforts that have attempted to posit the notion that an addictive personality might exist have done so by trying to identify the specific characteristics that are presumed to have become "rigid, habitual, and maladaptive." As such, many of these efforts appear to have been directed toward the formulation of a distinct personality disorder that can be associated with addiction. There are some problems with approaching this question in this manner. First, what are all the characteristics that combine to form a personality? Second, what and how many of these characteristics must be seen as being rigid, habitual, and maladaptive in order for a personality to be considered to be disordered? Third, and perhaps most importantly, how will these characteristics combine to predispose an individual to the addiction to mood-altering substances?

You can imagine that answering all of these questions would be a monumental undertaking. There will be no attempt to do so in this text. Nonetheless, it might be constructive to compare what we know about personalities to what we know about a person's genetic makeup, as was discussed in previous sections of this effort. We know that, as human beings, we all share some genetic characteristics in common. However, our genetics vary from individual to individual to combine in such a way as to make each individual unique in some way. No single individual shares exactly the same genetic makeup as another individual. This is true even for identical twins.

All that can be stated relative to genetics can also be stated in terms of an individual's personality. We may all share some common characteristics. But, these characteristics combine in such a way as to make each individual's personality unique and distinct from that of any other individual. The relative normalcy of an individual's expression of personality can only be assessed on a continuum that ranges from being more or less normal in terms of observed behavior to being extremely maladaptive in that the individual habitually behaves in ways that are self-defeating and/or harmful to others.

Just as it is unlikely that we can identify an addict by assuming there exists a specific genetic profile which predisposes an individual to become an addict, it is equally unlikely that we will ever be able to identify a personality profile which we can reliably refer to as being an addictive personality.

Does this imply that observations which indicate that addicted persons appear to exhibit certain common personality traits is merely a matter of coincidence, and therefore meaningless? I, personally, do not believe this to be true. I believe that understanding how an individual characteristically views him or herself as an individual, and how he or she interacts with and relates to the environment may be very important in understanding how and why the individual initially became involved in the use of mood-altering substances. This is not the same as saying that an individual's personality might have caused the onset of the substance use, or even that it might predispose the individual to addiction. It is simply an assertion to effect that a person's tendencies to express himself or herself through certain behaviors might provide us with some insight as to why the individual might be drawn toward the use of mood-altering substances. It may also provide us with some insight as to why the substances the individual uses becomes so important to the individual that he or she behaves as if he or she cannot live without it.

Psychoanalytic perspectives have not historically played a major role in understanding and treating addictions. It is, however, the perspective that has provided us with the basis for our modern conceptualization of what we commonly call personality. In recent years, several psychoanalytic thinkers have offered what can be considered to be important contributions to the understanding of substance abuse. Psychoanalysis is also a perspective that concerns itself with theories of motivation. Developing an understanding of what might motivate a person to use and abuse mood-altering substances certainly seems pertinent to developing an operational conceptualization of addiction. Such an understanding would certainly seem to be relevant to the development of treatments intended to assist individuals to replace their substance abusing behavior with more appropriate and constructive alternatives. We will briefly examine the contributions made by two psychoanalytic authors.

Leon Wurmser (1984) suggested that early traumatic experiences causing individuals to develop overly harsh and destructive superegos may be at the root of substance-abusing behavior. Such experiences as "unusually severe real exposure to violence, sexual seduction, and brutal abandonment, and/or of real unreliability, mendacity, betrayal, and abandonment, and/or of parental intrusiveness or secretiveness" (p. 253) lead to hostility to authority, rebelliousness, and defiance. These experiences may also lead an individual to develop a harshness of internal authority and doubts about one's basic worth. Wurmser quoted one of his patients as the patient spoke of experiencing "a shadowy feeling of massive guilt, almost of mythical proportions" (1985, p. 90).

According to Wurmser, drugs temporarily disable the threatening internal authority and neutralize the feelings of doubt and guilt within the individual. An unintentional effect of the drugs is that they not only disable the unwanted feelings and thoughts, but they severely limit other superego functions as well. Included among the undesirable effects of the drug use is that the internal stability of mood and affect, the ego-ideal, self-observation, understanding of the boundaries of outer reality and self-care (1984, p. 232) are negatively affected as well. This accounts for why patients present as being grandiose, avoidant, and manipulative, and they appear to be unaware of the dangers that might result from their behavior. In essence, Wurmser's assertion is that the use of drugs represents an "archaic, global" way to avoid the feelings and impulses of pain, anxiety, and shame which threatens the substance abuser.

To treat this condition, Wurmser places emphasis on the psychoanalytic analysis of the superego. He also favors "deeply grounded combination treatments" that include self-help groups, pharmacologic treatment, education, and family counseling (1985, p. 95).

Another author, Edward Khantzian (1980), proposed that deficits, not conflicts, underlie the substance abuser's problems. He suggested that weaknesses and inadequacies in the "ego" or "self" compel individuals to seek relief through the use of specific mood-altering substances. Khantzian, when speaking of opiate users, stated, "Our experience suggests that the problems with aggression in such individuals are in part a function of an excessive reservoir of intense affect—partly constitutional and partly environmental in origin—interacting with psychological (ego) structures which are underdeveloped or deficient and thus fail to contain such affect" (p. 35). Selectivity is one hallmark in this theory. That is, individuals seek the specific effects of specific drugs in an effort to escape their troublesome thoughts and feelings. For example, Khantzian asserts that cocaine abusers exhibit different ranges of predisposing factors that might include symptoms relating to dysthymic disorder, cocaine abstinence depression, hyperactivity/attention deficit disorder, or bipolar disorder (1984, p. 758). Khantzian (1985, 1997) refers to the use of drugs as an effort to "self-medicate." Addictive behaviors are often pursued in an expression of the panicked need to escape from affect-generated helplessness.

The treatment that Khantzian developed to alleviate these problems is referred to as Modified Dynamic Group Therapy (MDGT) (Khantzian et al., 1990). The MDGT effort targets affect-tolerance, the building of self-esteem, the discussion and improvement of interpersonal relationships, and the development of appropriate self-care strategies (McLellan et al., 1990).

While there are other psychoanalytic theories that attempt to explain substance abuse from a psychoanalytic perspective, the above-mentioned two have been most useful to me in understanding some of the problems I have observed in my patients. Also, the treatments recommended by these two authors directly target specific problems commonly exhibited by substance-dependent patients. Neither of these two theories attempts to propose that there exists one specific personality predisposing individuals to addiction.

Wurmser proposes that traumatic experiences during developmental years result in the development of an overly harsh superego (conscience) which, in turn, causes the individual to experience unbearable guilt and feelings of worthlessness. More than half of all substance-dependent patients I have worked with over the years reported histories wherein they experienced traumatic events which negatively effected their emotional, moral, and intellectual development. In these patients, guilt, shame, and feelings of worthlessness have been issues that have consistently required clinical attention in addition to the treatment of their addictions.

Khantzian's suggestion that substance abuse stems from a deficient or underdeveloped ego supports my own observations of patients over the years. As I had previously stated, I have never been able to associate substance-abusing behavior with any specific personality or characterological type. Still, almost all substance-dependent individuals exhibit behavior that is noticeably immature and indicative of an underdeveloped sense of self. Their behavior, in almost all cases, indicates that they are deficient in appropriate socialization, they exhibit very poor impulse control, and they exhibit an obvious inability to accurately interpret objective reality. Substance-dependent patients also tend to exhibit extreme self-centeredness, poor insight into their own behavior, and an inability to tolerate unpleasant thoughts and emotions. My observations of substance-dependent patients' common characteristics are very much in line with the characteristics (sociopathy, aggressiveness, impulsiveness, pleasure-seeking, defiance of authority, an inability to form stable and lasting relationships, etc.) identified by the PD and MAC scales on the MMPI as being predictive of potential substance abuse. Anyone who has ever worked with substance-dependent patients will tell you that these patients rely entirely on immature ego defenses, such as repression or denial, regression, projection, and displacement.

There is no personality type that can be consistently associated with addiction. We cannot say, for example, that all people who exhibit characteristics consistent with that of someone who appears to have a dependent personality, a borderline personality, or a sociopathic personality is likely to become an addict. Assuming that there exists an addictive personality is almost as harmful as assuming that addiction is a disease. It places all addicted persons under one conceptual umbrella. It assumes that they are all the same; therefore, addiction is the same problem for all.

This does not mean, however, that addicted persons are always characteristically dissimilar. On the contrary, it seems very apparent that addicted persons frequently exhibit some characteristics or personality traits that appear to be common among addicted persons as a group. Some exhibit more of these common characteristics; some exhibit fewer of these characteristics. No single addicted individual exhibits exactly the same set of traits or characteristics as another addicted individual. What this means is that even though addicted persons as a collective may share some characteristics or traits in common, each individual has a unique personality comprised of characteristics that are unique only to that individual.

Recently, there has been a suggestion that there might be a basis for assuming that the addicts exhibit certain characteristics so consistently that we might be able to define this constellation of characteristics as representing an "addictive character" (Johnson, 2002).

The author went so far as to offer DSM-style criteria for the identification of this specific character:

- Has a denial system that allows persistent engagement in addictive activity despite obvious harm of three (or more) of the following:
  * Responds with addictive activity when feeling helpless (includes engaging in the addictive activity when experiencing intolerance of affect)
  * Idealizes the addictive activity
  * Resorts to addictive activity in preference to interpersonal support
  * When engaged in a relationship and conflict arises, resorts to addictive activity in place of effective interpersonal communication

If the patient meets criteria for a personality disorder, the diagnosis is "addictive personality disorder." If the patient has a level of functioning above that of a personality disorder, the diagnosis is addictive character, neurotic level of functioning (p.143). Johnson goes on to offer a DSM-style set of criteria for determining physical addiction as well.

Personally, I believe that the criterion set forth within the DSM-IV (APA, 1994) adequately assists in identifying the various substance-dependence disorders. The possible value of Johnson's classification is that it allows the clinician the opportunity to consider the patient's problem in light of the patient's expression of certain personality characteristics. However, there are many characteristics exhibited by addicted persons which this particular conceptualization ignores, such as sociopathy, aggressiveness, pleasure-seeking, defiance of authority, etc. Additionally, assuming the possibility that limitations in the patients functioning might render this rather limited set of characteristics to be representative of a personality disorder severely restricts a working definition of what constitutes a personality. Individuals can suffer from any number of mental disorders which severely limit their ability to function without exhibiting symptoms associated with a personality disorder. Despite these criticisms, Johnson's proposition adds some depth and breadth toward operationally defining what a given patient might be experiencing when it is said that he or she suffers from a substance-dependence disorder.

Why is it so important that we attempt to create an operational conceptualization of a patient's substance use problems that would include an understanding of the individual's personality or characteristic style? It is important for several reasons. First, an individual's personality or characteristic style allows us to gain a glimpse of how the individual perceives himself or herself as an individual entity. Second, it allows us to obtain an image as to how the individual perceives himself or herself in relation to the world that surrounds the individual. Third, and perhaps most importantly, it helps us to better understand what might motivate the individual to engage in the type of behaviors that are causing the individual to experience problems. In essence, understanding the addicted person's personality allows us to see their problems from within a specific context, a context that is representative of their personal, individual experience of living. When this can be accomplished, the clinician understands that every individual's experience of substance dependence is unique to each individual.

When we can conceptualize the substance-dependent patient's problems in this manner we can, in turn, attempt to devise treatment strategies that have meaning and pertinence to the patient. This operational conceptualization almost always gives us a better chance of creating treatment plans that the patient will see as being relevant to his or her life; thereby creating a greater assurance that the patient will actively engage in the kinds of therapeutic activities that have the greatest potential of correcting the problems that he or she is experiencing.

Twelve-step treatment totally ignores the notion of individuality. An individual's personality has absolutely no meaning in twelve-step treatment. In fact, twelve-step doctrine goes to great lengths to diminish the importance of an individual's personality. Twelve-step treatment assumes that all patients are characteristically similar and all suffer from exactly the same problems. Perhaps, this is one reason that so many people who seek help by attending twelve-step programs simply quit going for help. They may believe that what they are being asked to do in the name of treatment has no real relevance to what they have been experiencing. There is the distinct possibility that most people actually value their individuality!

As we create an operational conceptualization of a patient's substance dependence, is there any need to go beyond obtaining a glimpse of the patient's personality or characteristic style? Yes, there is definitely a need to go a little further in developing insight into the patient's problem. While understanding the patient's personality traits provides us with a great deal of insight into how a given individual expresses what he or she is experiencing it does not tell us exactly what the individual is experiencing, or has experienced in the past.

Experience is what shapes our character, and our overall personality. Experiences, past and present, form the basis for how we think and feel about ourselves, how we interact with the world around us, and of how we see ourselves as fitting into that world. It is, therefore, very important that we learn as much as we possibly can about our patient's life history, from birth to the present time. It is particularly important that we gain knowledge of significant experiences and events that may have had a formative effect in the development of the patient's character or personality.

Wurmser and Khantzian apparently believed that the early experiences of substance-dependent persons are at the root of their current behavior. To review, Wurmser (1984) suggested that early traumatic experiences causing individuals to develop overly harsh and destructive superegos may be at the root of substance-abusing behavior. Khantzian (1980) suggested that weaknesses and inadequacies in the "ego" or "self" compel individuals to seek relief through the use of specific mood-altering substances. Wurmser sees early trauma as a potential cause for substance abuse. Khantzian sees that holes in the organization of the self—how the individual protects, regulates, cares for, and thinks of himself or herself—as being a potential cause for substance abuse.

In general, all personality theories place much emphasis on the role that experience plays in the development of individual personality and behavior. In a sense, individuals are more or less defined by their respective histories. Another presumption of most personality theories is that the behavior a person chooses to engage in serves an adaptive function representing a response to the experiences the person has endured—*all behavior serves a function.*

Yes, Wurmser and Khantzian, along with many other theorists, believe that substance use serves an adaptive and defensive function! For example, Wurmser believes that substance use is an attempt to alleviate the pressures emanating from an overly harsh superego. Khantzian sees the use of substances as a means to self-medicate to escape feelings of helplessness caused by holes and deficiencies existing within the ego.

No matter what theory, or what perspective, one would choose as a means to offer an explanation as why an individual might engage in the use of substances, at the basis of that theory you will see that the use of mood-altering substances serves a purpose for the individual. Of course, all existing theories also acknowledge that substance use is not an appropriate and constructive means of fulfilling individual needs.

Most peoples' initial experiences with alcohol or other mood-altering substances provide them with the sensation and perception that the substance fulfills their needs. It alleviates the pressures, or diminishes their discomfort, etc. Of course, the substance changes nothing for the individual other than it alters the person's thinking and perceptions to create the illusion that the substance is serving its purpose. Because the individual perceives that the substance is doing its job and because the individual lacks the skills or the means to find more appropriate and effective ways of fulfilling his or her needs or easing their discomfort, the individual becomes psychologically reliant on the substance. Over time, and with repeated use of the substance, this psychological reliance is reinforced, while physiological dependence may also become a concern. The person becomes stuck.

In consideration of all of the previous discussion, the following operational definition of substance dependence is offered:

> *Substance dependence represents a psychological, and sometimes physiological, reliance upon a given mood-altering substance that serves an adaptive and defensive function in response to a real or perceived need or an existing coping deficit for which the individual has not yet developed the specific skills or learned the appropriate functional behaviors needed to fulfill this need or to correct the deficit in a more effective and constructive manner. This reliance will result in the repetitious use of mood-altering substances that will endure until such time as the individual develops the skills or learns the appropriate behaviors needed to fulfill his or her need or correct an existing deficit in a more effective and constructive manner.*

Why is this a more accurate and realistic definition of addiction?

First of all, this definition does not assume that the substance-dependent person suffers from a disease. Although the definition does assume that substance use is rooted in underlying psychological pathology, that pathology can be defined in terms of an individual's personal development or the individual's lack of development.

Second, this definition places the individual's substance use in a context wherein the person's behavior can be seen as being purposeful. One basic assumption held to be true within the behavioral sciences, regardless of the theoretical perspective, is that behavior does not occur in a vacuum. There is always a reason that certain human beings engage in certain behaviors.

This definition allows for individual differences. Every individual develops a distinct personality which is expressed in terms of his or her uniquely individual behaviors. The individual's personality or character is based upon the experiences the individual has endured throughout his or her life. The behaviors that the individual chooses to engage in serve a function within the context of the individual's life experiences.

This definition does not assume that an individual will forever be dependent upon mood-altering substances. It does allow for the possibility that the individual will grow and acquire more constructive and functional behaviors as he or she matures. In fact, it implies that the individual will tend to learn and grow.

Lastly, and most importantly, this definition of substance dependence allows those who are given the responsibility of treating this behavior an opportunity to formulate an operational conceptualization of the individual patient's problem, which is meaningful to the individual and to the treatment provider; thereby, enabling the treatment provider with the means of designing treatment plans that are target specific and have the greatest potential for addressing the specific needs of that individual.

Thus far, we have examined the importance of accurate diagnosis. Diagnosis, although it is a very important step in the treatment process, is merely a starting point. Once a patient is identified as suffering from substance use disorder, it becomes extremely important to operationally define what that means for the patient. I described this defining process as being able to form an operational conceptualization of the patient's problems. We need to identify, as thoroughly as possible, those factors that might originate from within the patient, those factors which might originate from the patient's environment, and how the interaction between the patient and the environment contributes to the patient's substance-abusing behavior.

Understanding a patient's character or personality traits provides key insights as to why the patient engages in substance-using behavior. Substance use can be considered to serve an adaptive and defensive function for the patient when that behavior is viewed in the context of the patient's experiences and the effect that those

151

experiences might have on the development of the patient's character and personality. I believe these are the primary factors that originate within the individual that contribute to an individual's substance use problems.

How does the individual's environment contribute to substance-using behavior? When formulating an operational conceptualization of a patient's substance use disorder, it is always important to visualize how the patient's environment has contributed to the patient's problems. This can be tricky! It is tricky because environment is an ever-expanding construct. At birth, an individual's environment may consist of only the nuclear family. But, as the individual progresses in life, exposure to ever-expanding influences coming from a variety of new environmental contexts has the potential to impact the individual for better or for worse.

As much as the disease concept promoted by the adherents to twelve-step doctrine misidentifies those factors within the individual that are most likely to contribute to the development of addictions, it also fails to address how environmental factors might also contribute to the development of addictive behavior. Twelve-step promoters such as NCADD define addiction as a "primary, chronic disease with genetic, psychosocial, and environmental factors influencing its development and manifestations." However, little effort is ever spent in articulating how those "psychosocial" or "environmental factors" might influence individuals in ways that contribute to their addictions. For example, NCADD (2005) on its Web site states, "Substance abuse crosses all societal boundaries, affects both genders, every ethnic group, and people in every tax bracket." If substance abuse cannot be related to variations in societal contexts, gender, ethnicity, economic status, and so on, then to what influences are they referring? Is it simply that life on the planet Earth is conducive to the development of substance abuse problems? I do believe that more clarity is needed here, don't you?

NCADD also states, "Scientific documentation defines alcoholism and drug dependence as a disease that has roots in both genetic susceptibility and personal behavior" (Ibid.). Statements such as this place great emphasis on genetic susceptibility. Psychosocial factors are minimized when they are mislabeled as personal behavior.

Environmental influences are not even mentioned. The implication is that if one inherits the genetic disease of addiction, one is pretty much destined to become an addict despite one's social class, ethnicity, gender, and income potential.

Alcoholics Anonymous also has had little to say about how the environment effects the development of alcoholism. In fact, AA generally adopts the notion that alcoholism is a disease that transgresses all environmental boundaries. The Big Book states, "We are average Americans. All sections of the country and many of its occupations are represented, as well as many political, economic, social, and religious backgrounds" (p. 17).

Does the scientific documentation support such statements as that which is asserted by AA and NCADD? Not at all! Research certainly does not, in any way, support the notion that alcoholics, or any other group of substance abusers, are representative of the "average American."

While it may be argued that substance-abusing individuals can found to exist in all segments of American society, it doesn't necessarily follow that these individuals are represented equally. Existing research overwhelmingly indicates that some groups of people appear to produce many more substance-abusing persons than do others. The incidence of substance abuse and dependence is higher for those individuals that come from disadvantaged socioeconomic classes (Newcomb and Bentler, 1989; Hawkins et al., 1987). It has been demonstrated that the incidence of substance use and dependence is higher among specific minority groups (SAMSHA, 2003; Jones-Webb, et al., 1997; Wallace, 1999). Additionally, age appears to be related to substance abuse with the highest incidence of substance abuse occurring at approximately twenty-one years and slowly declining thereafter (SAMSHA, 2003).

While such environmental factors as poverty, ethnicity, age, and many others can be related to substance use and dependence, it cannot be stated definitively that these factors cause individuals to become involved in the use of alcohol or drugs. While research suggests that such environmental factors may play some role in the development of substance use, most individuals who can be described as being poor, young, or belonging to a specific minority population never abuse or become dependent upon alcohol or drugs.

The environmental factor most frequently associated with an individual's development of substance use disorders is that of the family environment. Family, in most cases, represents the most dominant influence in any individual's development. Many studies have examined how the family environment might contribute to an individual's substance abuse problems along a variety of family characteristics. As was cited in previous chapters, addiction appears to run in families. Family modeling of drug-abusing behavior and parental attitudes toward children's drug use are specifically related to the risk of alcohol and other drug abuse. Poor parenting practices, high levels of conflict in the family, and a low degree of bonding between children and parents appear to increase risk for adolescent problem behaviors generally, including the abuse of alcohol and other drugs (Hawkins et al., 1987; 1992).

Gaining insight into the substance-dependent patient's family history has always aided in my understanding of how and why the patient developed substance abuse problems. Very often, a patient's problems—substance use among others—are reflections of problems that have existed within the family environment throughout the patient's development.

In the last several years, I have been involved in the assessment of youth who have come into contact with the juvenile courts. For the most part, my role in the assessment of these youths was to screen them for possible substance abuse problems. I also conducted family assessments. Results of these assessments were used by the courts to make decisions as to what treatments would most likely be of benefit to the youth in question and/or to make decisions regarding placement of the youth. I would estimate that I have conducted hundreds of these assessments.

What I have observed is that, with rare exception, problems exhibited by the subject of these assessment efforts were similarly exhibited by one or both of the youth's parents. If the youth had siblings, they too would exhibit problems similar in nature to that of the parents. For example, if the youth who was the subject of the assessment effort was determined to suffer from a disorder related to depression, it was very likely that one or both of the youth's parents would also have experienced a history of problems related to depression.

One assessment outcome which came as a surprise to me was that even though the youth might be heavily involved in the abuse of mood-altering substances, the youth's parents frequently would not report histories of substance abuse or dependence. In most instances, even if the parents did report histories of substance abuse or dependence, the parental abuse of substances occurred prior to the birth of the subject. I would estimate that, overall, less than 30 percent of the youth diagnosed as suffering from a substance use disorder had parents with current or past histories of substance abuse. Only 3 percent of these children had parents who evidenced existing or recent problems related to substance use.

What I did find, consistently, was that within the families of these children there was almost always evidence of problems, such as poor parenting practices, high levels of conflict in the family, and a low degree of bonding between children and parents, along with a host of other family problems. Very often, one or both of the parents of these children could also be diagnosed as suffering from identifiable mental disorders for which they were in need of treatment.

In essence, what I observed was that if the parents did not possess the skills allowing them to effectively and appropriately deal with their own problems, the children were also limited in their abilities to deal with problems. Simply stated, these children suffered because their parents could not model, or otherwise impart, effective coping skills to their children. Within these families, the children who were drawn to the use and abuse of mood-altering substances engaged in such behavior because their use of these substances allowed them a form of escape from problems that they could not otherwise confront through the application of effective and constructive coping strategies.

Chapter One discussed how the observation that alcoholism, and other addictions, seems to run in families has been used to support the notion that addiction was a genetic disease. Yet, only 20 to 30 percent of children coming from homes wherein one or both parents suffered alcoholism ever develop problems relating to alcohol abuse.

Similar logic has been employed when looking at the environmental influences. It has frequently been asserted that growing up in a family environment wherein one or more parents engage in the use of alcohol or drugs greatly enhances the chances that a child will engage in the use of alcohol or other drugs. No doubt, there is some legitimacy to this observation. Children do, very frequently, imitate the behavior of their parents. It seems reasonable to assume that if a child's parents engage in the use of mood-altering substances as a means to escape troublesome thoughts and feelings, the child will also learn to deal with their thoughts and emotions in an equally dysfunctional manner. Additionally, growing up in an alcohol- and drug-influenced family environment has been associated with the development of many other mental problems as well.

What is surprising is that most children who grow up in families wherein parents suffer addictions do not always follow the examples offered to them by their parents. Whether you see family in terms of genetics or environmental influences, it really does appear that children who follow in the footsteps of their parents' addictions are the exception and not the rule. That's the good news.

According to the 2003 National Survey on Drug Use and Health (SAMSHA, 2003), about 10.9 million persons aged twelve to twenty reported drinking alcohol in the month prior to the survey interview in 2003 (29 percent of this age group). Nearly 7.2 million (19.2 percent) were binge drinkers, and 2.3 million (6.1 percent) were heavy drinkers. Illicit drug use among youths aged twelve to seventeen was 11.2 percent of those surveyed.

These figures do not significantly vary from the previous surveys that have been conducted in recent years. If one were to assume that either genetics or environmental influences absolutely predispose children to become alcohol or drug abusers, we would see a steady increase in the alcohol- and drug-use rates from year to year, and from generation to generation. For every generation, there would be exponential increases in the number of youth who become involved of alcohol or drugs. While we have observed increases over the years that these surveys have been conducted, we have not observed exponential or gigantic increases that would substantiate claims of predisposition.

As was stated, this is good news. The bad news is that, according to these SAMSHA surveys, our substance abuse problems do not appear to be getting significantly better either.

What does all this mean in terms of our ability to form an operational conceptualization of a substance-dependent patient's problems? Well, for me it simply underscores the relevance of understanding how the individual's environment has contributed to his or her substance use. Influences originating from within the patient's family environment play some role in the development of the patient's problem. It might well mean that the patient's family did model substance-abusing behavior, or the family suffered from other problems which contributed in some way to the patient's problems. It might mean that the patient's race or ethnicity influenced him or her in some way. It might mean that the patient's socioeconomic status has had some influence as well.

These environmental influences, in and of themselves, cannot be seen as sole determinants of the patient's behavior. It seems more than reasonable to assume that the environmental influences experienced by the individual patient did help to shape the character of the individual that presents for treatment of his or her substance use disorder. Understanding what role these influences might have had in the development of the patient's problems only serves to enhance the overall operational conceptualization of the patient with all the various factors that contributed to the problem that you are attempting to treat.

If the clinician can form an operational conceptualization of the patient's substance use disorder, which includes an understanding of the patient's personality and characteristic style of behavior, an understanding of the significant events and experiences that helped to shape the patient's current relationship to the world, and an understanding of the environmental forces that might have influenced the patient; a comprehensive image of the nature of the patient's substance use disorder begins to materialize. As that image materializes, it reveals, very often in operational and concrete terms, which factors most likely played a contributing role in the development of the patient's disorder.

Once the clinician has created this operational conceptualization, treatment strategies can be devised that specifically target the actual contributing factors. This allows the clinician the ability to devise a treatment plan for the individual patient to correct specific deficits, build specific skills, and learn more effective and constructive ways of relating to and interacting with his or her immediate environment.

> Don't existing treatment programs and facilities attempt to do this for their patients? The answer to this question, for the most part, would have to be NO.

While some treatment programs that utilize the twelve-step treatment approach might require their patients to undergo psychiatric or psychological exams, the primary purpose of these efforts is merely to screen their patients for coexisting disorders. If, or more appropriately when, patients are determined to suffer from problems in addition to their substance use disorders, these additional problems are most often treated separately, if at all..

Some existing programs may also go to the effort of conducting social histories (sometimes called psychosocial histories) of the patients. In most instances, these are merely used to verify a family history of substance use problems. In some instances, family counseling is offered. But usually, family counseling is minimal and primarily used to confront the patient regarding the patient's substance use. All other environmental influences revealed as a result of conducting a social history are generally ignored in twelve-step treatment.

In Chapter Five, twelve-step treatment was described in detail. This treatment approach assumes that all addicts suffer from the same ill-defined disease. According to adherents of this ideology, the ill-defined disease of addiction is incurable; it can only be arrested by a lifelong commitment to the *mystical* twelve-step path to recovery. Formal twelve-step treatment consists of having patients progress through the first four of the Twelve Steps of Alcoholics Anonymous. The act of progressing through steps in formal treatment consists primarily of admitting to powerlessness and insanity, abandonment of free will, and praying and pleading with God. Unfortunately, this approach simply does not work for most substance-dependent persons.

I hope you understand why twelve-step treatment doesn't work. Traditional understanding of addiction represents a gross misconceptualization of a very real mental disorder. This treatment approach fails to operationally define what it might be attempting to correct, and it fails to target any of the specific factors causing patients to become dependent on mood-altering substances. It's an approach that simply attempts to convince the patients that they must turn their life and their will over to God (as each patient might understand Him) and have faith that He will lead them in the right direction. All too often, it does this in exchange for great sums of money. I have always believed that to engage prayer or to develop a devotion to a specific faith should be pursuits that did not depend upon one's economic resources.

References

Chapter Seven

Alcoholics Anonymous. (1939). *The Story of How More than One Hundred Men Have Recovered from Alcoholism.* Works Publishing Company.

American Psychiatric Association. (1994). *Diagnostic and Statistical Manual of Mental Disorders, Fourth Edition.* (p. 181). Washington, DC.

Dodes, L. M. (2002). *The Heart of Addiction.* New York, NY: Harper Collins.

Dworetzky, J. P. (1982). *Psychology.* St. Paul, MN: West Publishing Company.

Hathaway, S. R., and McKinley, J. C. (1943). *Manual for the Minnesota Mutliphasic Personality Inventory.* New York, NY: Psychological Corporation.

Hawkins, J. D., Lishner, D. M., Jenson, J. M., and Catalano, R. F. (1987). Delinquents and drugs: What the evidence suggests about prevention and treatment programming. National Institute on Drug Abuse. (DHHS Publication No. ADM 87-1537). Washington, DC: U.S. Government Printing Office.

Hawkins, J. D., Catalano, R. F., and Miller, J. Y. (1992). Risk and protective factors for alcohol and other drug problems in adolescence and early adulthood: Implications for substance abuse prevention. *Psychological Bulletin,* **112(1)**, 64–105.

Hoffman, H., Loper, R. G., and Kammier, M. L. (1974). Identifying future alcoholics with MMPI alcoholism scores. *Quarterly Journal of Studies on Alcohol,* **35**, 490–498.

Johnson, B. (2002). Psychological addiction, physical addiction, addictive character, and addictive personality disorder: A nosology of addictive disorders. *Canadian Journal of Psychiatry*, **11(1)**, 135–160.

Jones-Webb, R., Snowden, L., Herd, D., Short, B., and Hannan, P. (1997). Alcohol related problems among Black, Hispanic, and White men: The contribution of neighborhood poverty. *Journal of Studies on Alcohol*, **58**, 539–545.

Khantzian, E. J. (1980). An ego-self theory of substance dependence. In D. J. Littieri, M. Sawyers, and H. W. Pearson (Eds.), *Theories of Addiction* (NIDA Research Monograph No. 30, DHHS Publication No. ADM 80-967). Washington, DC: U.S. Government Printing Office.

Khantzian, E. J. (1985). The self-medication hypothesis of addictive disorders: Focus on heroin and cocaine dependence. *American Journal of Psychiatry*, **142**, 1259–1264.

Khantzian, E. J. (1997). The self-medication hypothesis of substance use disorders: A reconsideration and recent application. *Harvard Review of Psychiatry*, **4**, 231–244.

Khantzian, E. J., and Khantzian, N. J. (1984). Cocaine addiction: Is there a psychological predisposition? *Psychiatric Annals*, **14(10)**, 753–759.

Khantzian, E. J., Halliday, K. S., and McAuliffe, W. E. (1990). *Addiction and the Vulnerable Self: Modified Dynamic Group Therapy for Substance Abusers*. New York, NY: Guilford Press.

Loper, R. G., Kammier, M. L., and Hoffman, H. (1973). MMPI characteristics of college freshman males who later became alcoholics. *Journal or Abnormal Psychology*, **82**, 159–162.

Ludwig, A. M. (1988). *Understanding the Alcoholics' Mind.* New York, NY: Oxford University Press.

MacAndrew, C. (1981). What the Mac Scale tells us about men alcoholics. *Journal of Studies on Alcohol,* **42**, 604–625.

MacAndrew, C. (1986a). Similarities in self-depiction of female alcoholics and psychiatric outpatients: Examination of Eysenck's dimension of emotionality in woman. *Journal of Studies on Alcohol,* **47**, 478–484.

MacAndrew, C. (1986b). Toward psychometric detection of substance misuse in young men: The SAP scale. *Journal of Studies on Alcohol,* **47**, 161–166.

McLellan, A. T., Woody, G. E., Luborsky, L., and O'Brien, C. P. (1990). Foreword.

In Khantzian, E. J., Halliday, K. S., and McAuliffe, W. E. (Eds.), *Addiction and the Vulnerable Self: Modified Dynamic Group Therapy for Substance Abusers.* New York, NY: Guilford Press.

Miessner, W. W. (1980). Theories of personality and psychopathology: Classical psychoanalysis. In H. I. Kaplan, A. M. Freedman, and B. J. Sadock (eds.), *Comprehensive Textbook of Psychiatry (3rd Ed.).* Baltimore, MD: Williams and Wilikns.

National Council on Alcoholism and Drug Dependence. (2005). Definition of alcoholism. Web site: http://www.ncadd.org/facts/defalc.html.

National Council on Alcoholism and Drug Dependence. (2005). Alcoholism and Drug Dependence are America's Number One Health Problem. Web site: http://www.ncadd.org/facts/numberoneproblem.html.

Newcomb, M. D., and Bentler, P. M. (1989). Substance use and abuse among children and teenagers. *American Psychologist,* **44**, 242–248.

Substance Abuse and Mental Health Services Administration. (2003). Prevalence of substance abuse among racial and ethnic subgroups in the U.S. Report incorporating results from the 1991–1993 National Household Surveys on Drug Abuse. Web site: http://www.drugabusestatistics.samhsa.gov/nhsda/ethnic/ethn1013.html.

Substance Abuse and Mental Health Services Administration. (2003). Overview of findings from the 2003 National Survey on Drug Use and Health. Department of Health and Human Services. Office of Applied Studies. Web site: http://www.oas.samhsa.gov/nhsda/2k3nsduh/2k3Overview.htm#toc.

Wallace, J. M. (1999). The social ecology of addiction: Race, risk and resilience. *Pediatrics,* **103(5)**, 1122–1127.

Wurmser, L. (1984). The role of superego conflicts in substance abuse and their treatment. *International Journal of Psychoanalytic Psychotherapy,* **10**, 227–258.

Wurmser, L. (1985). Denial and split identity: Timely issues in the psychoanalytic psychotherapy of compulsive drug users. *Journal of Substance Abuse Treatment,* **2**, 89–96.

Zucker, R. A., and Gomberg, E. S. L. (1986). Etiology of alcoholism reconsidered: The case for biopsychosocial process. *American Psychologist,* **41**, 783–793.

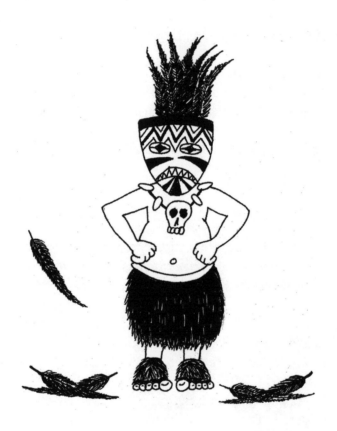

Chapter Eight

More Misdirection: The Myth of Dual Diagnosis

Any discussion relating to addiction would not be complete without making reference to the work of E. M. Jellinek. Jellinek devoted a great deal of time and effort to an extensive survey of Alcoholics Anonymous members prior to 1952. A summary of the observations that Jellinek had made as a result of his survey, entitled *Phases of Alcohol Addiction*, was published in 1952. Jellinek's work has frequently been cited in support of the notion that holds alcoholism to be a medical disease. However, when his writings are examined thoroughly, it seems clear that any support Jellinek might have offered to the mistaken notion that alcoholism is primarily a physical disease has been largely overstated.

In one section of that summary, Jellinek wrote: "In both groups (alcohol addicts and habitual symptomatic excessive drinkers) the excessive drinking is a symptom of underlying psychological or social pathology, but in one group after several years of excessive drinking 'loss of control' over the alcohol intake occurs, while in the other group this phenomenon never develops. The group with the loss of control is designated as 'alcohol addicts.'"

Jellinek identified two specific groups of problem drinkers, and the one group that exhibited a loss of control over their intake of alcohol he referred to as alcohol addicts. The remaining group, which Jellinek labeled habitual symptomatic excessive drinkers, appeared to maintain some control over their consumption of alcohol. In essence, Jellinek had stated that both of the groups of excessive drinkers exhibited apparent psychological and/or social problems. Jellinek stated that he considered the excessive drinking to be a symptom of those identifiable abnormal conditions.

Jellinek continued to describe his observations as follows:

> The "loss of control" is a disease condition per se which results from a process that superimposes itself upon those abnormal psychological conditions of which excessive drinking is a symptom.... Whether this superimposed process is of a psychological nature or whether some physical pathology is involved cannot be stated as yet with any degree of assurance, the claims of various investigators notwithstanding. Nor is it possible to go beyond conjecture concerning the question whether the "loss of control" originates in a predisposing factor (psychological or physical) or whether it is a factor acquired in the course of prolonged excessive drinking.

Jellinek stated that he believed the loss of control was a "disease condition," in itself, that occurred in addition to the existing abnormal psychological conditions that served as the underlying cause of the excessive drinking. Jellinek was careful to qualify this speculative statement by indicating that he could not determine if this "disease condition" could be attributed to psychological or physical factors, or whether it might simply be attributed to prolonged and repeated exposure to alcohol.

By the time that Jellinek's summary was published, Alcoholics Anonymous and other groups that promoted AA doctrine had long been asserting their belief that alcoholism was a physical disease. Despite the speculative nature of Jellinek's description to the effect that addiction appeared to be a disease process, these collective interests were very quick to pounce upon his work in support of their beliefs and their respective agendas. As Goodman and Levy (1997) wrote:

> A great deal of attention was paid to the medical and biochemical aspects of Jellinek's theoretical musings

regarding "alcohol addicts" by alcoholism counselors, Alcoholics Anonymous, and the National Council of Alcoholism. If alcoholism could be understood as primarily a medical disease then its victims could be considered medical patients worthy of treatment rather than condemnation. They would be able to get a better deal in terms of treatment and insurance coverage. The idea of alcoholics as "crazy people" was to be avoided and discredited at all costs.

It seems very clear that AA, NCA (now NCADD), and others chose to emphasize the mere speculation that addiction might be a disease, even though its etiology could not be determined in any way, in order to support their beliefs and their socio-economic agendas. If they could convince everyone that alcoholism was a medical disease, then alcoholics would receive better deals in terms of treatment and insurance coverage. Also, by ignoring Jellinek's more salient observations—that excessive drinking was symptomatic of underlying abnormal psychological conditions—they could avoid the stigma that was associated with mental illness.

As we now know, AA, NCADD, and other twelve-step promoters were very successful in their efforts to convey the notion that addiction is primarily a medical disease. In Chapter Four, we discussed the considerable influence that AA and other twelve-step promoters have had on the evolution of the addictions treatment industry. Today, more than 90 percent of the addictions treatment programs in the United States base their respective efforts on the mistaken and misguided belief that addiction to alcohol and other mood-altering substances is a medical disease that can only be successfully treated through the application of the twelve-step treatment model.

As successful as AA and other twelve-step promoters have been in advancing this mistaken belief, they have been equally successful in their efforts to discredit and avoid the idea that alcoholics, and other addicts, are crazy people. Their success is evidenced by the fact that addictive behavior is considered by most treatment professionals to be a primary disease etiologically rooted in genetics and biochemical processes, not a symptomatic expression of underlying mental illness.

Despite the fact that such assertions have literally no scientific support, more than 90 percent of all existing addiction treatment programs base their respective treatment efforts upon this untenable conceptualization. What makes this picture even more convoluted and illogical is that the overwhelming majority of these treatment efforts truly believe that the best way to treat this presumed medical disease is to convince their patients that they must adhere to a mystical form of treatment. Is it really any wonder why the most frequent outcome to this type of treatment is relapse?

Well then, if substance abuse disorders are not medical diseases caused by genetic and biochemical abnormalities, why do seemingly normal people persistently engage in such behaviors? The plain and simple truth is: they don't!

> Normal, happy, well-adjusted human beings do not engage in the persistent and habitual abuse of mood-altering chemicals!

By definition, the persistent and habitual use of mood-altering substances is abnormal behavior indicative of the existence of an abnormal psychological condition!

As was discussed in the previous chapter, all human behavior is purposeful. The only reason to use alcohol or any other mood-altering substance is as a means to an end. Addictive behavior simply does not occur from within a void. A normal human being doesn't simply wake up one morning and say, "I think I'll just go out and get drunk today, and maybe the next day as well." Thoughts, such as, "Perhaps, I'll go buy a bag of pot and smoke it all, and maybe try a bunch of other drugs," don't spontaneously pop into a person's mind, motivating and driving him or her to embark on a lifelong habit of substance use. An individual only uses alcohol or drugs because he or she anticipates and expects some sort of benefit or pay off as a result of the use of a given substance.

Let's use a simple example as a demonstration of this simple but obvious fact. Let's envision a young woman, whom we will call Eve, who is employed in a very fast-paced and demanding profession such as nursing. Eve and one of her coworkers decide to go out for a drink or two after they have both endured a long, arduous, and very busy shift at a local hospital. By modern standards of conduct, this would be considered to be relatively normal behavior to anyone observing Eve and her friend.

Eve has never been a big drinker. Usually, Eve doesn't profess to even like the taste of most alcoholic beverages. Eve has never kept any alcoholic beverages at home in her apartment.

On this occasion, Eve goes out for a couple of drinks, a seemingly innocuous activity. Eve notices that after she and her friend have indulged in this seemingly innocuous activity, she feels quite relaxed, and the tension that she was experiencing from her day at work seems but a distant memory. Usually, it takes several hours for Eve to begin to feel relaxed after a busy shift at the hospital. Eve thinks, *Hey, I guess it wouldn't hurt anything to have a drink or two now and then after work just to relax.* So, from that point on, Eve has one or two drinks almost every evening after her shift, just to relax.

Having a couple of drinks after work is not likely to become much of a problem for anyone, if that's the only time a person indulges in the use of alcohol. Still, are there other, perhaps better, ways for Eve to become relaxed? Certainly there are other more constructive ways to relax. Eve could stop at a gym each night after work for a short physical workout. Eve could learn yoga or some other form of meditation to relax. Eve could even go for a short, brisk walk to relax. There are many other activities in which Eve could engage that would allow her to achieve a state of relaxation. But, Eve perceives that having one or two drinks is the most expedient way for her to quickly and easily achieve a state of relaxation.

Now, if this is as far as Eve's drinking goes, her drinking is probably never going to become a serious problem for her. But, what if Eve is the type of person who has always found it difficult to relax and calm down? What if Eve begins to perceive that she needs to drink to relax on weekends, or when she interacts with others socially? Eve might even begin to believe that the only way she can relax is by having a few drinks.

Let us envision that Eve begins to drink every time she begins to feel the desire to relax. Eventually, Eve's drinking gradually increases to the point wherein she is drinking everyday, sometimes several times a day—just to relax. Sometimes, she needs more than one or two drinks to feel relaxed. Although, Eve might not have noticed, she doesn't feel relaxed until after she has consumed enough alcohol to become intoxicated. In fact, Eve's first innocuous single drink after work has escalated to several drinks daily. Eve's alcohol use might now be considered a problem.

Eve's story is not yet complete. Eve's supervisor at work has noticed that, on some days, Eve appears sluggish, as if she is hungover, and she has recently made mistakes with patients' medications. One day, Eve's supervisor believes that she detected the odor of alcohol on Eve's breath. The supervisor reports her observations to the appropriate authorities.

Ultimately, Eve is required to undergo assessment of and treatment for her alcohol problem. Eve is referred to a treatment program that holds employee assistance agreements with the nursing board in her home state. This treatment program is, naturally, a twelve-step program. The counselor assigned to Eve conducts his assessment of her alcohol problems and determines that Eve suffers from alcohol abuse, according to DSM-IV criteria. The counselor recommends that Eve should attend outpatient treatment for this disorder and she should also attend Alcoholics Anonymous, at least three times each week. Eve's outpatient treatment plan simply states that Eve will work through the first four steps of AA with her counselor and then commit to weekly attendance of AA. Eve agrees to this treatment. Eve is also given a one year probationary period by the nursing board.

During treatment, Eve complies with all that is asked of her. Eve also remains totally abstinent for a period of approximately ten months. But, then she begins to relapse—not so much that anybody would notice. Eve is able to hide her drinking behavior until she successfully completes her probationary period. Slowly then, Eve's drinking once again begins to escalate.

What went wrong here? Eve didn't have a long history of alcohol abuse. Her drinking appeared to simply just get out of hand. Eve completed twelve-step treatment, and she attended AA regularly, even after she relapsed. Why didn't this intervention work in Eve's case?

The most reasonable explanation for the failure of Eve's treatment is that the treatment recommended for Eve simply attempted to alleviate a symptom of an abnormal psychological condition. The overall goal of Eve's treatment was simply for her to achieve a state of abstinence, which she did for a time. However, Eve's alcohol use was actually an indication that she was experiencing an underlying problem for which she sought relief. Eve's alcohol use served a purpose. It provided her with a means to achieve a state of relaxation, or an escape from what Eve perceived to be unrelenting stress and tension. Eve, prior to her experience with alcohol, had never been able to find a reliable and efficient means of relaxing. Eve's treatment did not attempt to address this issue because, as far as her counselor was concerned, Eve's primary problem was that she drank too much; Eves' problems were rooted in the onset of a genetic and biochemical disease. According to her twelve-step counselor, the only way that Eve could ever overcome her problem was to "turn her life and her will over to God as she understood Him."

In Eve's case, her use of alcohol was symptomatic of an inability to find an effective and constructive way to rid herself of accumulating stress and tension, or find a way to relax. If we merely remove alcohol from her life, little has been accomplished. What we end up with is a sober person wracked with stress and tension who knows no effective and constructive means of escape. If Eve never finds a more effective and constructive way to cope with the many stressors in her life, sooner or later she will return to the only means she had found to be effective—alcohol use.

Although this is an overly simplistic hypothetical example, it does illustrate the basic principle that substance abuse is always "symptomatic of underlying abnormal psychological conditions." When a person engages in the abuse of a mood-altering substance, it should always be assumed that the use of that substance is serving a purpose. The substance use is a means to an end. The person engages in the persistent and habitual use of this substance because there is a benefit or pay-off. The common question is, "If it is true that people only abuse mood-altering substances because they are seeking escape from other underlying problems, why is it that so many people who are diagnosed with substance use disorders are never diagnosed as suffering from any other mental illness?"

The answer to that question is simple: no one is looking for other problems! As had been repeatedly noted, most of all existing treatment programs base their treatment efforts on the belief that substance abuse and dependence are primary medical diseases caused by genetic and biochemical abnormalities. For these programs, there is no reason to identify other problems that a patient might be experiencing. It is assumed that even if the patient does exhibit other apparent problems, these problems are not likely to be the cause of the patient's substance abuse. In most instances, if it is observed that patients in these twelve-step programs do exhibit symptoms associated with other mental illnesses, it is assumed that these symptoms are the result of the patients' substance use. All too often, it is also assumed that these symptoms will disappear if the patient abstains from the use of mood-altering substances. Unfortunately, this is not what happens with most patients.

Another explanation as to why most patients entering twelve-step treatment are not diagnosed as suffering from other identifiable mental problems is that the overwhelming majority of counselors working within these programs are not sufficiently trained to be capable of reliably identifying other problems. In fact, if the counselor assigned to a given patient is credentialed only to be a licensed or certified drug and alcohol counselor, he or she is not qualified to diagnose any problems other than a substance use disorder. This is true in all fifty states within our nation.

Am I saying that twelve-step treatment programs make no attempt to diagnose other problems that might be related a given patient's alcohol and/or drug use problems? For the most part, I would have to answer yes. Precious few programs require patients to undergo psychological evaluations, psychiatric examinations, or even medical examinations. Such extensive evaluation may only be required by some inpatient treatment programs. Even then, if it becomes apparent that a patient suffers from other mental disorders, these disorders are not generally treated during drug and alcohol treatment. Usually, these patients are referred to other agencies or programs for treatment after they complete their substance abuse program. If the patient is so impaired by the symptoms of another mental disorder that the patient is prohibited from competent participation in drug-and-alcohol treatment, that patient might be referred to another agency or program for stabilization prior to entering treatment for the substance use disorder.

The efforts of AA, addictions counselors, NCADD, and other twelve-step promoters to create the illusion that alcoholism and other addictions are primary medical diseases which are completely distinct and separate from other mental illnesses have been very effective. Over the last fifty years, these groups have convinced the general public, media, and governmental agencies that this scientifically unsupportable myth is the truth. Today, when someone is referred to as being an alcoholic or an addict, most people perceive this individual to be suffering from a disease over which the individual has little or no control. All too often, there is little thought given to the possibility that the individual is actually suffering from an abnormal psychological condition. The subsequent abuse of a mood-altering substance is merely one symptom of that condition.

Since addictions have been promoted as being distinct and wholly separate from other mental illnesses, efforts to devise treatment for addictions have also evolved in a manner completely separate from the treatment of other mental disorders. As Kenneth Gleaves (1996) wrote:

> In the United States, Alcoholics Anonymous (AA) and similar twelve-step groups have had almost complete reign over the substance abuse field and have either actively sought to have their views on addiction emphasized (primarily through the National Council on Alcoholism) or have passively allowed their programs to be incorporated into professional treatment settings which rely, in varying levels, upon twelve-step group involvement. It has been my experience (as a professional practitioner in the substance abuse/mental health field and as an educator involved in the training of substance abuse

counselors) that many recovering people feel their "life experience" of addiction and recovery through involvement with twelve-step groups in some way entitles them to forego the rigorous training demanded of professional counselors and therapists. Indeed, this belief often posits that one has "paid the dues" already and should be allowed to work with substance abusers by virtue of one's own recovery and knowledge of the twelve-step philosophy. Apart from the many professional and ethical concerns inherent in such an irrational approach to the substance abuse counseling field, there is a clear thread of logical inconsistency which frames this sort of thinking.

In essence, Gleaves is stating that twelve-step groups such as AA and the NCA, with their emphasis on the disease model of addiction, have had complete and total dominance in the addictions treatment field. He points out that, all too often, practitioners in the addictions treatment field believe that all they need to be effective in the provision of treatment to other substance abusers is their own "life experience" of recovery and their knowledge of twelve-step philosophy. Gleaves also points out that such an irrational approach to treatment raises many professional and ethical concerns.

Indeed, it is very clear that those who adhere to twelve-step philosophy have gone to great lengths to ensure alcoholics and other addicts are never to be regarded as being mentally ill. To avoid the stigma historically associated with mental illness and to overcome to beliefs that alcoholism and other addictions were caused by defects of character, adherents to the twelve-step philosophy purposely manufactured a perspective of addiction as a medical disease over which the afflicted individual had little control. Addiction was unlike any other mental or behavioral problem. This concept was promoted and nurtured until it became accepted wisdom. Accepted wisdom has convinced us that it is appropriate to treat what is presumed to be a genetic and biochemical disease using primarily undereducated, nonmedical personnel with personal histories replete with bad decisions. Even then, the only thing that resembles professional treatment in this scenario is the cost.

In 1985, J. R. Milam wrote, "After some fifteen years of surface conflict, the disease concept of alcoholism seems to have finally prevailed over the belief that that alcoholism is a symptom of a functional psychological disorder" (p.55). Milam continued, "Alcoholism is a unique field in which custom dictates that unsupported beliefs are more acceptable than hard data. In some areas, beliefs are so deeply entrenched that it is impossible to introduce factual knowledge at all" (p. 55). Today we have a large and growing alcoholism industry operating as though the disease has been defined and the treatment is known (Mulford, 1988). Almost everything that the American public believes to be scientific truth about alcoholism is false (Fingarette, 1989).

The authors cited above offer acutely accurate insight into the state of our current addictions treatment industry. The truth is the disease concept has been promoted so effectively and convincingly that 90 percent of the American public does agree with the proposition that alcoholism is a disease (Caetano, 1987). The addictions treatment industry does pretend that they, and only they, can treat the problem. The addictions treatment industry vehemently resists any scientific evidence which threatens the status quo. Finally, what AA and other twelve-step groups have promoted as the truth, and subsequently built upon in order to create our existing treatment industry is an absolute fabrication.

When Alcoholics Anonymous and other twelve-step promoters attempted to create distance between the phenomena of alcoholism and mental illness, they did so by selectively extracting only those findings and observations that would support their desire to portray the alcoholic as a victim of disease while choosing to ignore those that didn't. For example, referring to Jellinek's extensive survey and his subsequent observations, twelve-step groups extracted only those observations appearing to support their belief that alcoholism was a disease. They ignored and denied the obvious fact that Jellinek merely speculated that alcohol addicts appeared to suffer from a disease process which, at that point in time, could not be accurately defined. Today, that disease process still defies accurate definition according to any scientific or medical standard.

Through the manipulation and distortion of scientific findings over the course of many years, twelve-step promoters have been able to create an illusory image of alcoholism and addiction and sell this image to the American public. Alcoholics Anonymous and the various groups that support AA doctrine never actually defined alcoholism. They merely created the illusion that they understood alcoholism in a way that no one else could. Unfortunately, this is an illusion that is rife with falsehoods and glaring contradictions.

First, AA asserted, "We are average Americans" (Alcoholics Anonymous, p. 17). Despite this fundamental assertion, it is later stated that the alcoholic is "mentally and bodily different from his fellows" (p. 30). Which is it? Are alcoholics different from, or are they the same as the "average American"? It is also stated that alcoholics suffer from "a progressive illness. Over any considerable period we get worse, never better" (p. 30). But never fear for, "there is a solution.... When, therefore, we were approached by those in whom the problem had been solved, there was nothing left for us but to pick up the simple kit of spiritual tools laid at our feet. We have found much of heaven and we have been rocketed into a fourth dimension of existence of which we had not even dreamed" (p. 25). Wait a minute—did they say the problem had been solved? I thought it, the illness, "got worse, never better."

Boy, I'm confused. Aren't you?

Alcoholics Anonymous: *The Story of How More than One Hundred Men Have Recovered from Alcoholism* was first published in 1939. It is now on its fourth edition which was published in 2001. This book, which is frequently referred to as the Big Book, serves as the bible for those who adhere to AA's doctrine. AA's convoluted, contradictory, and contaminated description of alcoholism as it is laid out in this publication is the fountainhead of the illusory definition of addiction which 90 percent of the American public has come to accept as scientific fact! Even more terrifying is the fact that after seventy years, the sentimental rambling and mystical blarney contained in this book forms the theoretical foundation upon which our current addiction treatment industry was built! It's all illusion.

None of it has ever been supported by scientific evidence or by any other objective means.

E. Gordis (1987) offered a summary of his view of the state of the treatment of alcoholism as it has evolved into modern times:

> Yet in the case of alcoholism, our whole treatment system, with its innumerable therapies, armies of therapists, large and expensive programs, endless conferences, innovation and public relations activities is founded on hunch, not science. Contemporary treatment for alcoholism owes its existence more to historical processes than to science. Yet the history of medicine demonstrates repeatedly that unevaluated treatment, no matter how compassionately administered, is frequently useless and wasteful and sometimes dangerous and harmful. The lesson we have learned is that what is plausible may be false, and what is done sincerely may be useless or worse.

Dr. Gordis affirmed that our current system of treating alcoholism owed its existence to a historical tradition that was based on a hunch, not science. Despite the compassion and good intentions that may have initiated this tradition of treatment, it could be useless and even harmful to continue to employ these unevaluated traditional treatment practices.

As was illustrated earlier in this chapter, E. M. Jellinek's most specific observation was that excessive drinking is symptomatic of underlying abnormal psychological conditions. This was true in 1952. To date, this still remains as the most plausible explanation as to why individuals engage in the persistent and habitual use of mood-altering chemicals.

Although Jellinek may have been among the first to articulate an observed association between abnormal psychological conditions and substance use, there is an ever-expanding body of scientific theory and empirical evidence offering scientific support to his observations. Many empirical studies have established associations between abnormal psychological conditions and substance-abusing behavior. Some of this was outlined in Chapter Six.

That some relationship exists between other mental illness and substance abuse became very apparent when the results of the data from the Epidemiological Catchment Area study (Regier et al., 1990) indicated that 53 percent of individuals who have a lifetime diagnosis of a drug use disorder also have a lifetime diagnosis of a mental disorder. Actually, the results obtained from the ECA study were not really earth-shattering. As early as the 1960s and 1970s, researchers began to discover solid evidence indicating that individuals who suffer from substance abuse disorders very frequently also suffer from other identifiable mental illness. Early epidemiological studies reported that 25 to 50 percent of newly admitted psychiatric patients had concomitant drug- and/or alcohol-abuse problems (Simon, Epstein, and Reynolds, 1968; Crowley, Chesluk, Dilts, and Hart, 1974).

In 1967, Petrie offered a typology of alcoholics which asserted that some alcoholics were driven to drink to modulate the intensity of anxiety-producing stimuli. According to Petrie, without the use of alcohol, these anxiety-producing stimuli would be too painful and anxiety-provoking for these individuals to tolerate. Later research (Sher and Levinson, 1982) supported Petrie's assertions but the researchers qualified that support by stating that there appeared to be a special group of drinkers who may experience elevated or special kinds of anxiety.

Since then, associations between substance abuse and almost all forms of mental illness have been established. Substance abuse has been linked to serious and persistent mental illnesses, such as schizophrenia (Drake et al., 1990), all forms of anxiety disorders (Bowen et al., 1984; Schuckit, 1992), depressive disorders (Schuckit et al., 1997), personality disorders (Nace, 1989; Ekleberry, 1996), and so on.

With increasing evidence indicating the existence of some relationship between addictions and other mental illness, individuals who appeared to be suffering from a substance use disorder along with, or in addition to, other Axis I or Axis II disorders came to be referred to as being "dual diagnosis" patients. The National Mental Health Association (2005) on its Web site states, "The following psychiatric problems are common to occur in dual diagnosis—i.e., in tandem with alcohol or drug dependency: depressive disorders such as depression and bipolar disorder; anxiety disorders, including generalized anxiety disorder, panic disorder, obsessive-compulsive disorder, and phobias; other psychiatric disorders, such as schizophrenia and personality disorders."

The term dual diagnosis has become the new buzz word within the treatment industry. By 1989, the terms dual diagnosis and dual disorders (Minkoff and Drake, 1991; Evans and Sullivan, 1990) had become widely accepted as broad labels for patients that presented with both substance-related and mental health disorders. So dramatic has been the impact of this supposedly new and revolutionary concept that in 1992 the Substance Abuse and Mental Health Services Administration (SAMHSA) was created by congressional action and presidential signature. SAMHSA was created for the purpose of coordinating the efforts of the Center for Substance Abuse Prevention (CSAP), the Center for Substance Abuse Treatment (CSAT), and the Center for Mental Health Services (CMHS). The overall intent of this reorganization, of sorts, was to oversee strategies for improving services for persons with *co-occurring* substance abuse and mental health disorders (SAMHSA, 1997).

Is the discovery that some individuals suffer from a substance use disorder and other mental illness new and revolutionary in any way? Well, E. M. Jellinek didn't think so in 1952. In fact, it would seem that Jellinek's observations indicated that all alcohol abusers and addicts suffered from abnormal psychological conditions of which alcohol use was merely a symptom. Before Jellinek, Freud and other classical analysts found intrapsychic conflict aplenty in both active and recovering alcoholics. There is even evidence that suggests that Bill Wilson, co-founder of Alcoholics Anonymous, understood disturbances in the self as being central to the etiology of alcoholism. Wilson taught that remediation of these disturbances is the core of the rehabilitation of the alcoholic (Levin, 1987).

I can recall the first time that I became aware of this revolutionary and innovative concept which is called dual diagnosis. By the time I had read literature relative to the new dual diagnosis categorization of patients, I had been serving as the director of a treatment program for nearly three years. I can recall my exact thoughts: *Gee wiz! Now that we know this, it's really going to help us serve our patients.* I hope you recognize the sarcasm. Having twenty years of experience in the treatment of addictions, I can, with all the sincerity, seriousness, and honesty, state that if there actually exists an individual who suffers from a substance use disorder that does not also suffer from an identifiable, preexisting Axis I or Axis II mental condition, I have yet to meet him or her.

Even though I didn't see that the term dual diagnosis represented anything new, or even particularly helpful, to the treatment of addictions, I did feel that it was incumbent of me in my role as the director of an addictions treatment program to ensure that my treatment staff was kept informed into new concepts that relate to the treatment of addictions. So, I conveyed this new concept to my employees during a regular in-service training. The overwhelming response that I received back from my staff was to the effect of, "well, duh." Obviously, they didn't find this revelation to be all that startling or helpful either.

The truth is the coinage of the term dual diagnosis has offered nothing of real value to anyone attempting to help individuals to free themselves from the grips of a substance use disorder. We have always known that individuals who become involved in the persistent and habitual use of alcohol and other chemical substances do so because they are attempting, in some way, to escape other problems for which they know no other effective means of escape. That this is so has been repeatedly been demonstrated by the likes of E. M. Jellinek and many other noteworthy researchers.

The term dual diagnosis is simply just another mythical construct used to ensure that substance use disorders continue to be regarded as being somehow separate and distinct from other mental illnesses. This becomes clearly evident when it is considered that this term is only applied to those individuals who are determined to suffer from a substance use disorder and who are found to exhibit symptoms consistent with an additional Axis I or Axis II diagnosis, according to DSM IV criteria.

Anyone involved in the treatment of individuals that suffer from mental disorders will testify that it is not at all unusual to find that patients can frequently be diagnosed as suffering from more than one identifiable mental disorder. For example, it is common for individuals who suffer from an anxiety disorder, such as posttraumatic stress disorder, to also exhibit symptoms consistent with an additional diagnosis of a mood disorder. It is equally common for individuals who suffer from personality disorders (an Axis II diagnosis) to also exhibit symptoms indicating they suffer from an anxiety disorder and/ or a mood disorder (both of which are Axis I diagnoses). Yet, such individuals are never referred to as being dual diagnosis patients.

Most qualified clinicians recognize that patients can, and frequently do, suffer from more than one identifiable mental problem. When this occurs, experienced and adequately trained clinicians understand that there is likely to be some relationship between the symptoms that qualify their patients for multiple diagnoses. As such, they attempt to treat their patients by implementing a systematic treatment approach designed to target all of their patients' symptoms.

Now, one would think that with a growing awareness that substance use disorders and other mental illness can and frequently do occur together would result in improvements in the way that these dual diagnosis patients are treated for their respective illnesses. Sadly, this has not really been the case. To date, treatment for dual diagnosis patients has been approached through the implementation of three basic models of treatment.

The first and most common treatment model is called "serial treatment" (SAMHSA, 1997). In this approach, each one of the individual's diagnosed illnesses is treated one at a time in a serial manner. For example, if an individual is diagnosed as suffering from a mood disorder and is also suffering from alcohol dependence, it is likely that the individual will be first treated for alcohol dependence, and then the individual will be referred to another agency for treatment of the mood disorder.

Most often the alcohol dependence is treated through the application of a twelve-step model. Then the individual is referred to another agency that can provide more traditional mental health therapy to assist the individual in overcoming the symptoms associated with the mood disorder.

In this serial approach, the patient is frequently shuttled between two or more service providers. Often, there is disagreement between the various agencies as to which illness should be treated first and how these problems should best be treated. There is generally no coordination of services between these service providers. As a result of this lack of coordination, the respective service providers may provide contradictory or incompatible treatments. For example, one means of treating the individual's mood disorder might be to prescribe antidepressant medication to alleviate the patient's disturbing symptoms. Many twelve-step treatment programs prohibit patient use of such medication during treatment and the patient is encouraged to avoid the use of psychotropic medication even after prolonged abstention.

The second treatment approach is referred to as being "simultaneous or parallel treatment" (Ibid). This approach allows two separate agencies to provide treatment to the patient at the same time; each treating one disorder. In theory, the two agencies would coordinate their services by allowing for exchange of information related to respective treatment efforts to maximize the benefit to the patient. In practice, experience has indicated that even when separate agencies begin with the best of intentions, adequate exchange of information is frequently a problem. Additionally, this type of effort frequently suffers from the same problems as serial treatment. The two agencies may, at times, propose conflicting goals and objectives for the patients.

The third treatment approach is referred to as "integrated treatment" (Ibid). This approach attempts to offer simultaneous treatment of all the patients' disorders by an appropriately dually-trained clinician, or a unified treatment team. Sometimes, the treatment team members all work for the same agency, although it is not unusual for two agencies to collaborate in an effort to create a unified treatment team. It is the responsibility of the treatment team to devise a treatment approach that recognizes the interconnectedness and complexities of the patient's psychiatric symptoms and the patient's substance use.

While this later approach has proven to be much more effective in terms of positive outcomes for dual diagnosis patients (Drake et al., 1995), there are still many difficulties in the implementation of integrated treatment efforts, which include, but are not limited to, the following: 1) funding streams are still separated between mental health and substance abuse; 2) agency turf issues are still a problem; 3) legitimate differences in professional philosophies exist as to how to best proceed with treatment; and 4) treatment team staff may lack the minimum degree of cross-training needed to work together and understand each other's vocabulary and techniques.

As was exemplified earlier in this chapter and as is evidenced from the descriptions of the treatment approaches described above, there has always been a vast chasm between the mental health treatment industry and the substance abuse treatment industry. This is a distance seldom transversed by either faction. Substance abuse treatment professionals rarely concern themselves with issues and problems related to mental health issues other than alcohol and drug abuse. Mental health practitioners rarely attempt to treat substance use disorders because this has traditionally been the twelve-stepper's territory. To say that there are differences in treatment philosophies between these two factions is an understatement.

In part, the separation between these two treatment fields has been created and perpetuated by those promoting substance use disorders to be primary medical diseases caused by genetic and biochemical abnormalities, while denying that substance use is related to or caused by underlying psychological problems.

It is also true that mental health practitioners frequently avoid providing treatment to substance abusers because they believe that they are inadequately trained in issues relating to substance use, and they perceive substance-abusing patients to be difficult to treat.

In reviewing the research, it was evident that those investigators whose research efforts ultimately resulted in the coinage of the term dual diagnosis did recognize that relationships do exist between other mental illnesses and the development and perpetuation of substance-using behavior. Most of these investigations also called for the creation of treatment approaches that attempt to treat both the substance-using behavior and the other existing mental health problems via some form of an integrated treatment. Some efforts have been made toward devising integrated treatment approaches.

Unfortunately, this remains the exception and not the rule in the treatment of those patients who are referred to as dual diagnosis patients. Osher (1996) described our nation's current treatment situation very accurately: "With empirical research and clinical experience supporting the effectiveness of integrated approaches, the time has come to reconsider the systematic division of addictive and mental health services. A change toward integrated system of care is likely to benefit the mental health addiction treatment needs of all people, not just those with co-occurring disorders."

It is extremely unfortunate that little has changed from 1996 to the present. Even though there has been much talk of the dual diagnosis patient, co-occurring disorders, integrated treatment, and such, there has been very little progress made in any effort to bridge the gap existing between the mental health professions and the addictions treatment industry. Even though SAMHSA was created in 1992 to guide an integration of mental health and substance use treatment programs, very little progress can be claimed. As it remains to this very day, the chasm between the mental health treatment industry and the substance abuse treatment industry remains as wide and impassible as ever.

At this point, I would be surprised if the reader is not more than just a little confused as to what the point of this chapter actually is. On the one hand, I have stated that the creation of the term dual diagnosis is yet another myth. On the other hand, I have gone to great lengths to demonstrate that individuals do, indeed, suffer from both substance use disorders and other mental illnesses. This does seem to be a glaring contradiction. Please allow me to explain my thinking here.

I consider the creation of the term dual diagnosis, at least as it has been popularly promoted, to be misleading in many respects. The creation of such a term attempts to convey the perception that, in some way or manner, new information has been discovered. This simply is not so. There have always been people who suffer from mental illness in addition to substance use problems. In fact, it has been known for many years that substance-using behavior is symptomatic of underlying psychological problems. Freud asserted this to be true; Jellinek explicitly stated that he observed this to be true; and many other theorists and empirical investigators have demonstrated the validity of this concept. The dual diagnosis patient has been the patient who has shown up in our treatment centers and psychiatric hospitals all along.

The term dual diagnosis has been misused from its inception. We do not refer to individuals suffering from more than one mental disorder as being dual diagnosis patients, even though such a descriptive term might be appropriate if it were applied equally to all. This term is only applied to those individuals who suffer from a substance use disorder and another identifiable Axis I or Axis II mental disorder. What such usage of this term does, in effect, is to perpetuate the notion that substance use disorders are in some form or manner distinct and separate from all other mental disorders. In essence, it attempts merely to preserve the integrity of the myth that substance use is the result of genetic and biochemical disease, and substance abuse is in no way related to other mental problems.

The term dual diagnosis has done nothing to bridge the gap between the substance abuse treatment industry and the mental health professions. Since the term implies a special consideration for individuals who suffer from substance abuse disorders, it has simply served as a way to maintain the status quo. It has merely served as a means for each side to maintain their stand firmly on the professional turf or territory for which they have each laid claim.

To state it very bluntly, the term dual diagnosis has been used as just more misdirection in an effort to maintain the mythical status of addiction as a disease.

References

Chapter Eight

Alcoholics Anonymous. (2001). *The Story of How More than One Hundred Men Have Recovered from Alcoholism. Fourth edition.* (pp. xxvii, 17, 18, 25, and 30). New York, NY: Alcoholics Anonymous World Services, Inc.

Bowen, R. C., Cipywych, D., D'Arcy, C., and Keegan, D. (1984). Alcoholism, anxiety disorder and agoraphobia. *Alcohol Clinical Experimental Research*, **8**, 48–50.

Caetano, R. (1987). Public opinions about alcoholism and its treatment. *Journal of Studies on Alcohol,* **48**, 153–160.

Crowley, T. J., Chesluk, D., Dilts, S., and Hart, R. (1974). Drug and Alcohol Abuse Among Psychiatric Admissions. *Archives of General Psychiatry*, **30**, 13–20.

Drake, R. E., Osher, F. C., Noorsday, D. L., Hurlbut, S. C., Teague, G. B., and Beaudett, M. S. (1990). Diagnosis of alcohol use disorders in schizophrenia. *Schizophrenic Bulletin I*, **16**, 57–67.

Drake, R. E., Noorsday, D. L., and Ackerson, T., (1995). Integrating mental health and substance abuse treatment. Lehman and Dickson, (Eds.), *Double Jeopardy: Chronic Mental Illness and Substance Use Disorders* (251-264). Chur, Switzerland: Harwood Academic Publishers.

Ekleberry, S. (1996) Dual diagnosis: Addiction and axis II personality disorders. *The Counselor,* March/April, 7–13.

Evans, K., and Sullivan, J. M. (1990). *Dual Diagnosis: Counseling the Mentally Ill Substance Abuser.* New York, NY: Guilford Press.

Fingarette, H. (1989). *Heavy Drinking: The Myth of Alcoholism as a Disease* (p. 1). Berkley, CA: University of California Press.

Gleaves, K. A. (1996). Clarifying the dichotomy between the 12-step approach and professional psychotherapy and counseling. *Journal of Rational Recovery,* **9(2),** Nov.–Dec.

Goodman, S., and Levy, S. J. (1997). The biopsychosocial model revisited: A psychodynamic view of addiction. Web site: http://www.rocklandpysch.com/biopsychosocial.htm.

Gordis, E. (1987). Accessible and affordable health care for alcoholism and related problems. *Journal of Studies on Alcohol,* **48,** 579–585.

Jellinek, E. M. (1952). Phases of alcohol addiction. *Quarterly Journal of Studies on Alcohol,* **13(4),** 673–684.

Milam, J. R. (1985). Disease concept of alcoholism. *Alcoholism and Addiction: The National Magazine,* **5(6),** 55.

Minkoff, K., and Drake, R. E. (1991). Dual Diagnosis of Major Mental Illness and Substance Disorder. *New Directions for Mental Health Services,* No. 50. San Francisco, CA: Jossey-Bass.

Mulford, H. (1988). Enhancing natural control of drinking behavior: Catching up with common sense. *Contemporary Drug Problems,* Fall, 321–334.

Nace, E. P. (1989). Substance use disorders and personality disorders: Comorbidity. *The Psychiatric Hospital,* **20(2),** 65–69.

National Mental Health Association. (2005). Substance Abuse-Dual Diagnosis Fact Sheet. Web site: http://www.nmha.org/infoctr/factsheets/03.cfm.

Petrie, A. (1967). *Individuality in Pain and Suffering.* Chicago, IL: University of Chicago Press.

Regier, D., Farmer, M. E., Rae, D. S., Locke, B. Z., Keith, S. J., Judd, L. L., and Goodwin, F. K. (1990). Comorbidity of mental disorders with alcohol and other drug abuse. Results from the Epidemiological Catchment Area (ECA) study. *Journal of the American Medical Association*, **264**, 2511–2518.

Schuckit, M. A. (1992). Anxiety disorders and substance abuse. Tasman, A., and Riba, B. R., (Eds.), *APA Annual Review of Psychiatry* (Vol. 11, 402–417). New York: American Psychiatric Press.

Schuckit, M. S., Tipp, J. E., Bergman, M., Reich, W., Hesselbrock, V. M., and Smith, T. L. (1997). Comparison of induced and independent major depressive disorder in 2,945 alcoholics. *American Journal of Psychiatry*, **126**, 39–46.

Sher, K. J. and Levinson, R. W. (1982). Risk for alcoholism and individual differences in stress response dampening effect of alcohol. *Journal of Abnormal Psychology*, **91**, 350–367.

Simon, A., Epstein, L. J., and Reynolds, L. (1968). Alcoholism in the Geriatric Mentally Ill. *Geriatrics*, **23(10)**, 125–131.

Substance Abuse and Mental Health Services Administration Advisory Council. (1997).

Improving Services for Individuals as Risk of, or With, Co-Occuring Substance Related and Mental Health Disorder. A SAMHSA Conference Report and a National Strategy. Rockville, MD: U.S. Department of Health and Human Services.

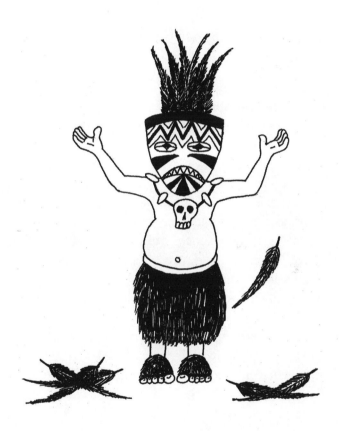

Chapter Nine

Understanding Addiction for What It Is

The noted contemporary psychologist, Albert Ellis (1973), has stated that human beings have an inborn tendency to disturb themselves and prolong their emotional dysfunctioning by holding on to irrational beliefs. According to Ellis, one of the ways in which we human beings perpetuate our misery is that we tend to "awfulize" what we perceive and what we experience. That is, our tendency as human beings is to embellish our perceptions and experiences in such a way as to make us believe that these experiences are more horrible or complicated than they really are. In short, we tend to make mountains out of molehills. This is certainly exemplified in our historical attempts to explain and understand the phenomenon of addiction as being a disease.

One of the first attempts to portray alcoholism as a disease was asserted by Dr. Benjamin Rush in the early 1800s. Rush believed that the overindulgence in alcohol, lying, murder, and political dissent were all diseases (Levine, 1978). Rush also believed that being a black person was a disease symptom (Szasz, 1977). According to Rush, individuals became drunkards because their "desire overpowered the will." In more modern terms, this simply means that people lost control over their drinking because they were morally weak. Rush's cure for this disease was temperance, meaning no hard liquor and only beer and wine in moderation (Ragge, 2002).

Rush's basic ideas held as the dominant view of alcoholism well into the early twentieth century, while his ideas formed the rationale for the various temperance movements from the early 1800s until Prohibition. The underlying message conveyed by the various temperance movements was that alcohol, especially in the form of distilled spirits, was "evil" and that anyone who would choose to indulge in the use of alcohol, even in moderation, would eventually become enslaved by alcohol. For those who supported the temperance movements, alcohol was seen as the root to all evil.

In essence, from the early 1800s up through the repeal of Prohibition in 1930, alcoholism was believed to be a disease characterized by some form of moral and/or spiritual weakness. Giving in to the temptation to use the "evil" alcohol was considered to be sinful, an alignment with the devil that would ultimately lead one to a life of sloth and continuing moral decline. Of course, the only cure to this disease was for the inebriate to give up alcohol completely, to confess one's sins, to pray for absolution of one's sins, and to vow to follow a Godly path from that point forward.

In 1939, Alcoholics Anonymous (AA) published its first edition of the Big Book. AA offered a somewhat different explanation of addiction to alcohol. The primary explanation was that alcoholics represent a select group of individuals who suffer from an inability to control their drinking from birth. This inability is explained in terms of their being born with a specific "allergy" (p. xxvii). Since these individuals are born with this inbred disease, it is considered to be irreversible. As such, it is believed that individuals who are born with this inbred allergy can never recover fully from this disease; it can only be controlled through complete abstinence. Of course, abstinence can only be achieved and maintained by following the spiritual guidance offered by the Twelve Steps outlined by AA.

Almost two centuries ago, it was proposed that overindulgence in the use of alcohol was a disease which was primarily characterized by some sort of moral weakness. This was essentially the popular view of alcoholism up through the 1930s when AA offered its explanation that asserted that alcoholism was a disease which was, in some manner, like an allergy. AA further asserted that individuals were born with this disease, and they could never rid themselves of this disease completely.

Throughout the nineteenth century and on into the early twentieth century, it was believed that the only way to overcome the disease of alcoholism was for the inebriate to give up alcohol completely, to confess one's sins, to pray for absolution of one's sins, and to vow to follow a godly path from that point forward. Then along came AA with its Twelve Steps that told us that the only way to control the disease of alcoholism was to ... now, wait just a minute! Do my eyes deceive me? Yes, I believe that AA's Twelve Steps told us, essentially, that the only way to control this inborn allergy was to give up alcohol completely, to confess one's sins, to pray for absolution of one's sins, and to vow to follow a godly path from that point forward! Oh, wait. I forgot one other important concept conveyed by AA's Twelve Steps; the AA message must also be passed on to others.

After seven decades, there is yet another explanation of addiction which has gained popularity within the last two decades. This model of addiction is referred to as the "biopsychosocial model" (Donovan and Marlatt, 1988). According to these researchers, addiction is impacted by physiological, behavioral, and environmental factors. This model holds that biological factors, such as a possible hereditary predisposition and/or altered brain chemistry, combine with an individual's desire to escape psychological discomfort through the use of alcohol and other drugs, and that this alcohol and drug use is reinforced by certain social interactions and conditions such as poverty, lack of employment, and family dysfunction.

Many researchers and clinical practitioners favor the biopsychosocial model because it offers a more holistic explanation of addiction. In essence, it offers a synthesis of the popular biological, psychological, and sociological explanations of addiction.

The biopsychosocial model also suggests that singular treatment efforts are unlikely to be sufficient to overcome addiction. Since the etiology of addiction is seen as a reinforcing interplay of factors from three spheres (bio, psycho, social) of existence, treatment for addiction should be designed to represent integrated efforts attempting to address the entire range of the afflicted individual's needs.

I agree with some of the basic tenants of the biopsychosocial model. I agree that it is important to attempt to formulate a conceptualization of a patient's substance abuse problem that considers the biological problems the patient incurs resulting from substance use. I agree that it is important to identify and operationalize the psychological and social factors that might have contributed to a patient's substance use problems. I also agree with the suggestion that treatment of a patient's substance use problems should be designed to address all of the various factors contributing to the patient's substance use problems. In short, I agree with this model's suggestion that treatment of addiction should be undertaken in a holistic manner.

Still, as an explanation of addiction, this model has many shortcomings. First, it still holds that addiction is a disease rooted in genetics and neurobiological abnormalities. As has been outlined in previous chapters, evidence that supports this belief is severely lacking. Second, and perhaps most importantly, this model fails to make any clear distinctions between what is causal of alcohol and/or drug use and what is consequential to substance use.

To say that addiction is a biopsychosocial phenomenon is really meaningless. If addiction is a biopsychosocial phenomenon, then I would have to ask what malady, illness, or disorder is not a biopsychosocial phenomenon? If one suffers from depression, are there not factors both within the individual and the environment which contributed to the problem? Is the individual not affected biologically, psychologically, and socially by the suffering of depression? Even if an individual suffers from common influenza, isn't it likely that biological agents from the environment interacted with physical vulnerabilities to cause the illness? When one is physically ill, does he or she not suffer psychologically and socially as well?

Human beings are creatures that exist biologically, psychologically, and socially all at the same time. There are constant interactions and interdependence between these spheres of human existence. There is no human experience than cannot be considered to be a biopsychosocial phenomenon! To say that addiction, specifically, is a biopsychosocial phenomenon is merely an exercise in semantics. It's just biopsychosocial babble!

To this point, we have seen how attempts to explain addiction have evolved over the last two centuries. Addiction has been explained as a disease caused by a moral and/or spiritual weakness. These beliefs seem even more ludicrous when it is considered that alcohol was seen as an instrument of the the devil. Addiction has been explained as a disease resembling an allergy of some sort. In more recent years, addiction has been explained to be a biopsychosocial phenomenon.

Do these explanations offer us a realistic way to understand addiction, or do these explanations make addiction more unique and mysterious than it really is? I believe these attempts to explain addiction, whether they are examined separately or collectively, represent irrational and overly general explanations of addiction which actually awfulize the problem.

Physiological dependence upon any mood-altering chemical substance can be explained much more simply and understandably. Addiction is not caused by a disease.

> Addiction is not the result of genetic or bio-chemical abnormalities existent in select individuals. All human beings can become physiologically dependent upon mood-altering chemical substances if used in sufficient amounts for a sufficient period of time.

Addiction is the predictable result of prolonged use of mood-altering chemical substances.

Addiction, when explained in simple biological terms, is no mystery. What happens to any individual human being when that individual consumes alcohol? Why does an individual become physiologically dependent upon alcohol when it is consumed on a persistent and prolonged basis? What can be stated about alcohol can also be considered to be true of any other mood-altering chemical.

First, let us take a look at the chemical properties of alcohol. Alcohol can be found in many forms. Most of the forms of alcohol cannot be ingested by human beings. To do so would be lethal. The only form of alcohol that can be ingested safely by humans is ethyl alcohol or ethanol. The chemical formula of ethanol is C2-H5-O-H. Ethanol is a chemical compound that is of a relatively small molecular size. It is perfectly soluble in water and is also soluble, to a lesser degree, in fat.

Ethanol is produced by the fermentation of sugar by enzymes contained in the microorganism yeast. Fermentation is a process that occurs naturally as yeast spores settle in the juices contained in fruits, some grains, and some vegetables. For example, wine is most often the result of the fermentation of grapes. Wine can also be made from tomatoes, dandelions, assorted berries, and so on. Beer is the result of the fermentation of malt to which hops are added as a flavoring.

It seems likely that man discovered ethyl alcohol (from this point on, alcohol will mean ethyl alcohol) by chance. That is, many years ago one of our ancestors ate fruit or consumed fruit juices that had fermented. Once this happened, the rest is, shall we say, history. Almost every human culture developed some way to produce alcohol by intentionally fermenting various fruits, grains, or vegetables. In time, man learned how to distill alcohol. Distillation is simply a way to remove the water from fermented products. When a product is distilled, it creates a higher concentration of alcohol within the fermented product. Brandy, bourbon, vodka, and sake are all examples of distilled alcohol.

Because of its small molecular size, alcohol does not require digestion to be absorbed into almost every cell within the human body. In fact, only a very small percentage of the alcohol ingested is completely digested. Approximately 20 percent of ingested alcohol is absorbed in the stomach while most of the remaining eighty percent is absorbed in the small intestine. Only a very small proportion of the alcohol ever descends further down the digestive tract.

Once absorbed, alcohol enters the bloodstream where it is transported to every cell in the body. Because of its small molecular size and its solubility, alcohol is able to cross the cell membranes of all the cells within the body in its unaltered state. This is the primary reason that alcohol is able to cause the widespread kinds of damage to the various organs within the body. It is very important to understand that once ingested, alcohol affects every cell within the human body.

Although our entire body is affected when we consume alcohol, its influence is most readily observed in terms of how alcohol affects our brain and the entire central nervous system (CNS). Alcohol is considered to be a central nervous system depressant. Alcohol also has other pharmaceutical properties. Alcohol's influence is very similar to other sedative-hypnotic drugs such as valium, barbiturates, and even general anesthetics.

When alcohol enters the cells within the CNS, it acts to inhibit or depress the normal neurotransmission processes within the brain. It first affects the inhibitory synapses of the brain. Since this serves a paradoxical influence in our experience of alcohol (depression of the inhibitory synapses), the first sensation a human being experiences as result of ingesting alcohol is a sensation of stimulation. Alcohol has, at times, been misclassified as being a stimulant. However, this stimulation sensation is caused by the depression of synaptic transmission of these inhibitory systems. The initial effects of alcohol cause humans to experience a reduction of anxiety, particularly in individuals who are prone toward feeling anxious, and feelings of euphoria.

Eventually, alcohol also begins to depress the excitatory systems within the brain. At this point, the subjective behavioral experience of alcohol, which is stimulative, catches up with the actual pharmacological effect, which is depressive.

Alcohol is addictive because the drinker develops a tolerance to alcohol, and the drinker subsequently requires more alcohol to experience the same effect experienced as a result of the initial exposure to alcohol. To understand this process of addiction, we must look at how the cells in the brain respond to the presence of alcohol.

Looking at the effect of alcohol on a cellular level, we must understand that all cells perform a function. This function is accomplished through metabolic processes undertaken by each individual cell. Any substance that enters through a cell's membrane is essentially treated as food or fuel for the natural metabolism of the cell. As was previously indicated, alcohol acts as a depressant. It is also a toxic substance. In short, alcohol is a poison. Even though alcohol easily enters almost all cells within the human body as a toxic and depressive substance, the respective cells still attempt to utilize it as fuel to create energy through metabolic processes.

When alcohol enters a cell, the cell has only two possible alternatives in response to the presence of alcohol. First, since alcohol is toxic in sufficient quantities, the cell can be damaged or destroyed by the presence of alcohol. Usually beginning drinkers do not ingest enough alcohol to cause widespread destruction of cells. However, it is important to consider that even when alcohol is ingested in moderation it causes damage and destroys some cells. When alcohol is ingested in sufficiently large quantities, it becomes lethal to human beings. Death is usually the result of alcohol's depression of the systems within the brain that control respiration (breathing).

The second, and for our purposes the more interesting, alternative is that the cell adapts to the presence of alcohol. The cell continues to attempt to function normally despite the presence of a toxic substance. Since alcohol depresses the functioning of all cells, it affects the overall functioning of every cell. However, the cells that are not damaged or destroyed adapt to the presence of alcohol. It is this adaptation response that causes tolerance to alcohol. Despite the presence of a poisonous substance, the cell adapts as best it can and attempts to continue to carry out its normal function. However, because alcohol is a depressant, some cells do not function as effectively and efficiently as they might under more normal conditions.

This tolerance, or cellular adaptation, to the presence of alcohol is what causes human beings to ingest more and more alcohol over time in an effort to experience the same effect that resulted from the initial exposure to alcohol. Cellular adaptation is also what causes us to experience withdrawal when alcohol is no longer present within the cells of our bodies. Cells adapt to the presence of alcohol and they attempt to carry out their normal function as best they can. Since the cell adapts its functioning in the presence of alcohol, it also has to adjust to the absence of alcohol. This adjustment, or adaptation, to the absence of alcohol also alters the function of most cells. Since alcohol serves as a depressant there is a rebound effect when alcohol becomes absent in the cell. The cell reacts to the absence of alcohol by becoming overactive. This is most apparent in the central nervous system, but it occurs in other body cells as well. This adaptation to the absence of alcohol accounts for the hangover human beings experience after a period of heavy drinking. We feel dysphoric, lethargic, and shaky when we experience what is commonly called a hangover. The headache that most people experience during a hangover is caused by a sudden reoxygenation of our brain cells, since alcohol acts to deplete cells of oxygen. A hangover is simply the result of our body cells making the attempt to return to normal functioning when alcohol leaves our bodies. We can stop the experience of a hangover by simply ingesting alcohol again.

Withdrawal can be understood as a massive, complicated hangover. Withdrawal occurs because the central nervous system becomes less sensitive to the effects of alcohol; it becomes tolerant of alcohol because the cells within the central nervous system adapt to alcohol's presence. This tolerance causes the individual to drink more and more alcohol in order to experience its effect. The more an individual drinks, the more the body attempts to accommodate to the presence of alcohol. When the individual ceases drinking and alcohol begins to leave the body, it causes the individual to experience the uncomfortable sensations because the cells must again adapt to a changing environment. In many instances, experienced drinkers resume their drinking to avoid the unpleasant and often dramatic consequences of withdrawal. This outlines the basic mechanics of physiological dependence. The defining hallmark of addiction to any substance is that the individual experiences withdrawal when they cease their use of that substance.

There is much more to this process than is explained here. Alcohol affects different systems within the body in different ways which serve to complicate this process. For example, over time and with prolonged exposure to alcohol, the liver begins to metabolize alcohol much faster than it normally would. When this occurs, it causes an increase in the liver's production of certain enzymes causing the individual to become less tolerant of alcohol, overall. This is why some chronic alcoholics appear to lose their tolerance to alcohol.

Alcohol affects all the cells within the body. Over time and with repeated exposure to alcohol, cells are damaged and destroyed to the extent that the normal functioning of all organic systems within the body are altered in some way.

Although this is a very simplified explanation of the process of addiction, this offers significant insight into the basic mechanics of physiological addiction. This is a process that will occur in all human beings who engage in prolonged and repeated overuse of alcohol and/or other chemical substances. It does not apply just to a select few. It applies to all. All human beings can become physiologically dependent upon any variety of chemical substances if they use enough of a given substance over a prolonged period of time.

Just how much exposure to alcohol, or any other chemical substance, it takes to bring about physiological dependence varies from individual to individual. It is likely that there are many variables unique to the individual that determine the point at which physiological dependence occurs. Variables likely to play a role in determining when and how an individual becomes physiologically dependent are likely to include body size and weight, metabolic rates, and other factors related to the overall functioning of the human body. Although many of these factors are, indeed, determined in part by individuals' genetic makeup, there is no evidence that one specific genetic type of individual is more prone to chemical dependency. Simply, all human beings can become physiologically dependent upon a given chemical substance if they experience repeated and prolonged exposure to that substance.

Keep in mind we are, at this point, talking about physiological addiction. Psychological addiction is a different matter which will be more specifically addressed later.

As was outlined in Chapter Five, there is only one way to overcome physiological dependence upon alcohol or any other drug. That is to endure the detoxification process and allow the cells within the body to return to a normal state of functioning without the presence of alcohol or other addictive chemical substances. The cure for physiological dependence upon any given substance is to discontinue the use of that substance.

Most people who become physiologically dependent upon alcohol or other drugs typically do not want to discontinue this use because this causes them to experience withdrawal. The symptoms of withdrawal cause physical and psychological discomfort ranging from very mild to very extreme, depending upon the specific drug used and the extent of the drug use. Individuals who have comparatively used more of a specific chemical over a greater period of time tend to experience more extreme symptoms during withdrawal.

Withdrawal from alcohol can be very dangerous, and it is sometimes difficult to predict the symptoms a given individual might experience. Mild symptoms can occur just after a few days of steady drinking. More serious symptoms generally do not occur until an individual has consumed the equivalent of a pint of whiskey (ten mixed drinks) per day for a period of ten days (Butz, 1982). Withdrawal symptoms can begin to manifest several hours to several days after the last drink. Symptoms tend to peak between the second and fourth day after the cessation of drinking and taper off within a week.

Three stages of withdrawal, of progressively greater severity, are generally recognized; although, most withdrawals do not progress to the third stage (Levin, 1987). During the first stage, the individual may experience tremulousness, restlessness, insomnia, loss of appetite, anxiety, and apprehensiveness, and pulse and respiration may become rapid as well. In the overwhelming majority of cases, withdrawal does not progress beyond this stage. While these symptoms can be extremely uncomfortable to the individual, they are not usually dangerous. The real danger is that the individual may want to drink to relieve their symptoms, which of course happens with great regularity.

If withdrawal progresses to the second stage, symptoms intensify: tremors become more severe; pulse, respiration, and blood pressure continue to elevate; and anxiety and apprehension may become more unbearable. The individual may also experience audio and/or visual hallucinations during this stage as well. These hallucinations are not an indication of psychotic disorder such as schizophrenia; they are purely a physiological phenomenon related to the individual's withdrawal. Even though the individual may be experiencing these hallucinations, he or she generally remains oriented to person, place, and time. It can, however, be very frightening for the individual.

The third stage of withdrawal is frequently referred to as delirium tremens (DTs). Relatively speaking, only a minority of alcoholics experience the severe and dangerous symptoms associated with this stage of withdrawal. In this stage, the alcoholic experiences abject terror. The individual's hallucinations become much more vivid and take on unusual forms wherein the individual might see crawling insects and strange animals (like the legendary pink elephant), and the hallucinations may include tactile sensations associated with the visual experiences. Pulse, respiration, and blood pressure may continue to rise. The individual may experience severe confusion and paranoia and lose all contact with reality. Fatalities are not uncommon during this stage of withdrawal from alcohol due to extreme physiological stress.

> Withdrawal from alcohol can be unpredictable and even life threatening in its most severe form. It really is no mystery why chronic alcoholics fear and avoid withdrawal.

Due to the potential danger associated with second and third stage withdrawal, all persons undergoing detoxification should do so only under the supervision of a qualified physician. Even in the initial stage of withdrawal, serious complications can occur due to other existing illnesses or organic damage caused by abuse of alcohol and/or other chemicals.

There are two primary types of programs which assist in detoxification: medical detoxification and social detoxification. Most often, medical detoxification programs are housed within hospitals or similar clinical settings. These medical detoxification programs are frequently inpatient programs requiring the patient to remain under medical supervision from a few days to several weeks depending upon the severity of withdrawal.

Social detoxification programs are also usually inpatient programs. However, there may or may not be medical personnel on-site at all times. Very often social detoxification programs offer introduction to twelve-step treatments in addition to providing a safe environment to endure the process of withdrawal. Social detoxification programs should be reserved for those who are expected to experience only mild withdrawal symptoms and suffer only minor organic impairment.

To the best of my knowledge, all states require that all licensed detoxification programs, even social detoxification programs, should be able to provide immediate access to medical assistance in the event that such assistance is required.

Most detoxification programs require patients to undergo medical examinations either prior to or upon admittance. This exam is necessary to identify and treat any medical problems as well as to determine how those problems might complicate the detoxification. Prolonged use of alcohol and/or other drugs causes organic damage. For those with many years of repeated and prolonged use of alcohol and other drugs, such damage in itself can be life threatening.

In these modern times, withdrawal can be medically treated to minimize the discomfort experienced. Often physicians prescribe medications such as Librium and Valium to minimize the anxiety and apprehension experienced during withdrawal. Physicians may also prescribe neuroleptic drugs to prevent seizures. Nutrition is also a concern. Frequently, detox patients are given vitamins, other nutritional supplements, and special diets to offset the self-inflicted physical abuse and neglect.

Detoxification, the medical treatment of withdrawal, represents the only major contribution that medical science has offered to the overall treatment of addiction. While this is significant and necessary to ensure the safety and well-being of alcoholics and other chemically dependent persons, it is just the beginning of the treatment process. Once the chemically dependent person has gone through withdrawal, much must be done to ensure that he or she does not return to the use of alcohol or other drugs.

After cessation of withdrawal symptoms, the physiological dependence upon alcohol or other drugs has, in all practical terms, been cured. Once the individual's body returns to a more normal state of functioning without the presence of alcohol or other drugs, he or she can no longer be considered physiologically dependent upon a given substance.

Logically, it would be assumed that enduring the symptoms of withdrawal, especially second and third stage symptoms, would deter an individual from wanting to use alcohol or other addicting substances again. Unfortunately, many individuals endure withdrawal only to return to the habitual use of substances and become physiologically dependent yet again. In fact, this happens with great regularity. It is obvious that there remains some compelling motivation which causes a return to the exact behavior that prompted the individual to become physically dependent in the first place.

Detoxification is only an initial step in the overall treatment of addiction. Although detoxification definitively resolves the issue of physiological dependence on mood-altering substances, it remains obvious that many individuals require additional treatment targeting other factors that have contributed to their dependence on mood-altering substances to avoid their eventual return to substance-abusing behavior.

References

Chapter Nine

Alcoholics Anonymous. (2001). *The Story of How More than One Hundred Men Have Recovered from Alcoholism. Fourth edition.* New York, NY: Alcoholics Anonymous World Services, Inc.

Butz, R. (1982). Intoxication and withdrawal. *Alcoholism: Development, Consequences, and Interventions*, 2nd Ed., N. J. Estes and M. E. Heinemann, (Eds.), (pp. 102–108). St. Louis, MO: C.V. Mosby.

Donovan, D. M., and Marlatt, G. A. (1988). *Assessment of Addictive Disorders.* New York, NY: Guilford Press.

Ellis, A. (1973). *Humanistic Psychotherapy: The Rational Emotive Approach.* New York, NY: McGraw-Hill.

Ellis, A. (1995). *The Essence of Rational Emotive Behavior Therapy.* Revised May 1994. Web site: http://www.rebt.ws/REBT%20 explained.htm.

Levine, H. G. (1978). The discovery of addiction: changing conceptions of habitual drunkenness in America. *Journal of Studies on Alcohol,* **39,** 143–174.

Levin, J. D. (1987). *Treatment of Alcoholism and Other Addictions: A Self-Psychology Approach.* (p. 25) Northvale, NJ: Jason Aronson, Inc.

Ragge, K. (2002). *More Revealed: A Critical Analysis of Alcoholics Anonymous and the Twelve Steps. Website: www.morerevealed. com/library/index.jsp.*

Szasz, T. S. (1977). *The Manufacture of Madness.* New York, NY: Harper & Row.

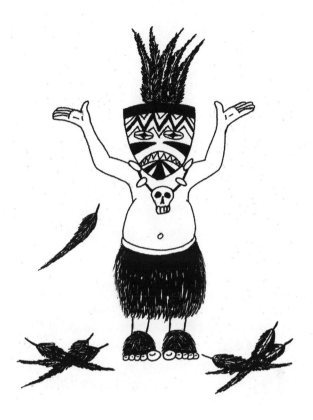

Chapter Ten

Understanding Psychological Dependence

In the previous chapter, physiological dependence was discussed to illustrate that addiction can be understood in simple biological terms. Any human being can become physiologically dependent upon alcohol and/or other drugs if these substances are used in sufficient quantities over a period of time. While it may be true that an individual's genetic makeup may play a minor role in the development of physiological dependence—genetics, in part, determine the individual's metabolic rate, height, weight, and other factors relating to the individual's overall bodily functioning—there is no evidence of a specific genetic type prone to physiological addiction. Physiological dependence is a predictable outcome to the persistent and prolonged use of alcohol or other drugs.

Also discussed was how physiological dependence upon alcohol and other drugs can be medically treated. This treatment is known as detoxification. Once an individual has completely experienced the detoxification process, he or she can no longer be considered to be physiologically dependent. In other words, physiological dependence is curable. It is not a lifelong phenomenon as it has frequently been portrayed.

However, a high percentage of those individuals who overcome a physiological dependence do return to the use of alcohol and/ or drugs. Many become physiologically dependent upon the same substances again. Considering that the withdrawal from alcohol and other substances is an unpleasant and sometimes a life-threatening experience, the big question which remains is: what would compel anyone to ever risk engaging in the use of an addictive substance once that person has overcome physiological dependence?

The answer should be obvious.

The compelling motivation that causes a return to the use of drugs or alcohol after experiencing withdrawal is that the individual was not only physically dependent but also psychologically dependent.

The individual will resume the use of mood-altering substances because of a perceived need to use a given substance in order to cope with life on a psychological level.

The DSM-IV (APA, 1994) provides for diagnosis of substance dependence disorders as being with physiological dependence or without physiological dependence. The implication is that individuals can be seen as being psychologically dependent upon a given substance even though they may not exhibit any indication of suffering from a physical dependence. There exists a presumption among clinicians that psychological dependence upon any given substance precedes the onset of physiological dependence.

It can be argued that there is a possibility an individual can become physiologically dependent upon a chemical substance without ever having become psychologically dependent. While, in theory, it might be possible, I have never observed such an occurrence in the twenty years that I have been involved in the treatment fields. Even in instances where an individual has become physiologically dependent upon legally prescribed and medically monitored medications (which happens much more frequently than most medical professionals will admit), psychological dependence is usually evident. In every instance I have encountered, there has been evidence indicating that the individual in question had experienced a psychological dependence upon the given substance long before exhibiting any behavioral indications of physical addiction.

We have already discussed detoxification, or the medical treatment of physiological dependence. While this form of treatment may or may not be accomplished within the context of a more general treatment approach, it has not historically been considered a significant aspect of treatment for chemical dependency. Most established treatment programs require that an individual should be detoxified prior to admittance into what we have traditionally called "substance use treatment." However, detoxification is separate and distinct from the traditional treatment of chemical dependency. Frequently, detoxification and traditional treatment of chemical dependency is accomplished in separate facilities, or at the very least, in separate units within a larger treatment facility.

When we speak of treatment of chemical dependency, we are referring primarily to the treatment of an individual's psychological dependence upon a given mood-altering chemical. Historically, this has consisted of an application of some form of twelve-step treatment. This model of treatment has been employed for the last seventy years. Twelve-step treatment is still utilized in more than 90 percent of all existing treatment programs despite the fact that it has never proven to be effective in any demonstrable way.

If our traditional means of treating psychological dependence upon mood-altering chemicals is ineffective, what should we do to more effectively assist individuals in their efforts to overcome their reliance upon these chemicals?

I believe that the first step in devising a more effective means of treating psychological dependence is to abandon the scientifically unsupportable notion that addiction to mood-altering chemicals is the result of disease. Our adherence to this blatant falsehood has done nothing to further our collective understanding of addictions, nor has it ever contributed anything toward making the treatment for these disorders more effective, or efficient.

Next, it is my belief that we must accept the evidence offered by such researchers as E. M. Jellinek (1952) and many other scientists. We must accept that all individuals who abuse alcohol and other drugs do suffer from "abnormal psychological conditions of which excessive drinking (and the use of other drugs) is a symptom."

By accepting that the excessive use of alcohol or other drugs is symptomatic of underlying abnormal psychological conditions, we can see that to effectively and definitively treat psychological dependence upon chemical substances we must move beyond the traditional goal of treatment. The only objective goal of traditional twelve-step treatment is to move the substance-abusing individual to abstinence. If this is all that can be accomplished with traditional treatment, we have done nothing for the affected individual except to remove the most obvious symptom of the disorder. We have actually done little, if anything, to address the problem(s) causing the individual's reliance on the mood-altering substances.

Taking this one step further along this line of logic; have we actually done anything significantly helpful to an individual whose only treatment has been directed toward the solitary goal of achieving abstinence? Achieving abstinence removes a serious threat to the individual's overall physical and mental health. Certainly this is a positive outcome; is it not? Of course it is! If this singular outcome were achieved in even a significant portion of these cases, we might have something to celebrate. Unfortunately, what we have learned is that the most frequent outcome of traditional treatment is not lifelong abstinence. The most predictable outcome of traditional twelve-step treatment has been, and still is, relapse.

Remember, that *all behavior, both functional and dysfunctional, serves a purpose.* No matter which scientific perspective is used to understand substance abuse disorders, it cannot be denied that, for better or worse, an individual's use of a mood-altering substance does serve a purpose.

If you will recall the hypothetical case example of Eve, her use of alcohol served a purpose in her life. For Eve, the use of alcohol provided her with a means of achieving a state of relaxation. Eve had never developed an efficient or effective means of achieving this desired state before she discovered that this relaxed state could be reliably achieved by her use of alcohol. Eve learned to rely upon alcohol to feel relaxed. This is a simplified example of psychological dependence.

Although Eve was merely diagnosed as suffering from alcohol abuse, her relapse after receiving outpatient twelve-step treatment, even with ongoing attendance of AA, clearly illustrated that she was dependent upon alcohol. Eve returned to the use of alcohol despite having full knowledge of the personal and social problems she experienced as a result of her alcohol use. On a psychological level, Eve came to depend upon alcohol.

Eve returned to the use of alcohol for several reasons. Eve was misdiagnosed. This is understandable because it is difficult, if not impossible, to effectively make a clear distinction between abuse and dependence. However, it seems likely that the failure to make this diagnostic distinction could account for Eve's relapse. Regardless of whether or not Eve had been accurately diagnosed, there was at least a 90 percent chance that Eve would be offered an ineffective treatment. Whether Eve had been diagnosed as being an alcohol abuser, alcohol dependent, or alcohol dependent with physiological dependence, there was a 90 percent probability that Eve would have been prescribed essentially the same treatment.

As it was, this probability was played out. Eve was ordered to attend a twelve-step treatment program. In treatment, Eve was taught that she had a genetic condition that caused her affinity to alcohol. She was also taught that the only way she could ever hope to be free of her alcohol use was to follow the Twelve Steps and attend Alcoholics Anonymous. Like so many others who have received this type of treatment, within a period of less than one year, Eve was using alcohol almost to the same extent that she had prior to treatment.

Eve was treated as though she was the victim of a genetic and/or biochemical disorder over which she had no control. Her only hope for recovery was to "turn her life and her will over to God as she understood Him" (Alcoholics Anonymous, 2001). The most plausible explanation as to why Eve relapsed is that she was offered a form of treatment that was not relevant, in any way, to the problem she was experiencing.

Eve learned to rely on alcohol to achieve relaxation. Eve knew no other way to achieve that state. During her treatment and in her subsequent attendance of AA, there was no acknowledgement that Eve's alcohol use served a purpose in her life. She was never offered any guidance or instruction as to how she might learn to achieve her goal of becoming relaxed in a more appropriate and constructive manner. Eve simply returned to the only behavior that had accomplished the desired goal of becoming relaxed. If Eve had been provided a more effective and constructive alternative to her use of alcohol, she might not have needed or desired to return to that use.

In Chapter 7, the following definition of substance dependence was offered:

Substance dependence represents a psychological, and sometimes physiological, reliance upon a given mood-altering substance that serves an adaptive and defensive function in response to a real or perceived need, or an existing coping deficit, for which the individual has not yet developed the specific skills or learned the appropriate functional behaviors needed to fulfill this need, or to correct the deficit in a more effective and constructive manner. This reliance will result in the repetitious use of mood-altering substances that will endure until such time as the individual develops the skills or learns the appropriate behaviors needed to fulfill his or her need, or correct an existing deficit in a more effective and constructive manner.

This definition is offered once again as means of adding clarity to our discussion of psychological dependence. Let us review Eve's case with this definition in mind to see if we can understand Eve's alcohol use in a more realistic and pragmatic manner.

As we have discussed with Eve's case, it seems clear that Eve became psychologically reliant upon alcohol. We have no evidence suggesting that Eve became physiologically dependent upon alcohol, as she exhibited no symptoms of withdrawal. On the surface, Eve appeared to be doing well since she abstained from alcohol use for a period of ten months. Despite appearances, she once again had an inability to achieve a state of relaxation. This symptom predates the onset of Eve's alcohol use, and therefore cannot be seen as a result of her alcohol use.

Did Eve's use of alcohol serve an adaptive or defensive function in her life? Clearly, it did. It provided Eve with a means of achieving a state of being that, for whatever reason, had previously not been available to her.

Was Eve's use of alcohol a response to a real or perceived need? Again, clearly it was. In Eve's case, she was never able to find an effective and easy way to relax prior to her discovery that this could be achieved simply by consuming alcohol. As we all know, we must be able to relax. No one can endure the ever-present stresses associated with modern living without occasionally taking some time to relax and let go.

Did Eve's reliance upon alcohol persist? Obviously, it did. Eve continued to rely on alcohol as evidenced by her relapse after only ten months. She returned to the only behavior that effectively achieved a state of relaxation. Relaxation was the goal of Eve's behavior; achieving that relaxed stated was the pay-off for using alcohol.

Now the pressing question is: *why* did Eve remain reliant upon alcohol?

Eve was told she suffered from a genetic and biochemical disease causing her to crave and rely upon alcohol. According to this line of thinking, there was no reason to encourage Eve to acquire new skills or to learn more appropriate and constructive behaviors. All she had to do was abstain from alcohol. After all, acquiring skills and learning new behaviors is certainly not going to alter one's genetics or reverse abnormal biochemical processes. Only God can do that! So, Eve was told she must "turn her life and her will over to God as she understood Him" (AA, Step 3). Then, Eve was told to she must continue to make "steps" until she became "entirely ready to have God remove all these defects" (AA, Step 7). Eve then had to "humbly ask Him to remove her shortcomings" (AA, p. 59, Step 8).

But, this didn't work! Within just months of committing to these sacred steps, Eve was once again relying upon alcohol. Did God forsake Eve? Did she not take these steps in earnest and with sufficient sincerity? Did this treatment fail because Eve didn't believe enough?

Can you imagine what this must have been like for Eve? She was led into believing that she suffered from some sort of indefinable genetic or biochemical disorder. She learned that if she asked humbly, God had the power to intervene and remove these defects from her life so that she could lead a normal existence. Unfortunately, Eve never sensed any kind of response or experienced any noticeable changes. Poor Eve! Despite her best and most sincere efforts, she was not only stressed and unable to relax, she was forsaken by God as well.

Can you imagine how one might be affected by this experience? The overwhelming majority of individuals, like Eve, experience this feeling of utter failure, abandonment, and disillusionment as a result of having invested themselves in such a misguided treatment.

As I have repeatedly stated, I do believe in God. I adhere to the Christian faith. I do believe that God and Christ positively influence our lives. But in all my religious studies, I have never been led to believe that God intervenes in our lives in such a manner as implied within the Twelve Steps of AA. Alternatively, I have learned that God gives us free will, giving each of us the ability to make decisions regarding our existence, for better or for worse. He also allows us to endure the consequences of our decisions, for better or for worse. God doesn't restore us to perfection in our earthly life. He encourages us to endure our imperfections on earth so that we appreciate what might be given to us when we place our faith in Him. Above all, God does not do for us that which He has given us the capacity to do for ourselves.

What might have saved Eve from relapse? What would have prevented her from feeling the guilt and shame that might come from her failure, and from feeling that she has been forsaken by God? If someone had offered Eve the opportunity to learn new skills or taught her that there were more effective and constructive ways to achieve a state of relaxation then she might not have had to rely upon alcohol. I do think that this alternative might have been worth a try, don't you?

The case of Eve is a hypothetical construct devised to illustrate some important points. But there is truth behind this hypothetical construct named Eve. I have seen many Eves. As unfortunate as it might be, all too many stories of twelve-step treatment have ended just as the case offered herein was portrayed.

Eve's case is oversimplified. I have seen few cases wherein it appeared as though an individual developed a dependence upon a chemical substance simply because of an inability to relax. With that said, I also have to state that I have seen hundreds of cases *wherein it appeared* that an inability to relax did lead an individual to turn to alcohol or some other drug to aid him or her in achieving a state of relaxation. Seems like a huge contradiction, does it not? Well, let me explain.

When an individual cannot relax, there is usually something much more complex (psychologically speaking) going on under the surface. Restlessness, uneasiness, hypervigilance, and other similar symptomology can be caused by a variety of identifiable psychological disorders and other problems. A few identifiable psychological disorders that present with these symptoms would include such disorders as depression (in its various forms), anxiety disorders, such as posttraumatic stress disorder, generalized anxiety disorder, and phobias, adjustment disorders, and more. Even situational problems, such as bereavement and relational problems, can be the cause of an inability to relax. With any of these disorders or problems, individuals can and do frequently turn to the use of alcohol and other drugs to help them relax or cope. It is not unusual to find that some of these individuals learn to rely upon these chemicals as a means of alleviating these undesirable symptoms.

That is my point. People do not just spontaneously begin to abuse alcohol and/or other drugs. *There is always a reason people engage in the use and abuse of alcohol or other drugs.* It is not because they are in some manner genetically or biochemically defective. As odd as it may sound, substance-using behavior is purposeful. It is certainly not appropriate and constructive behavior. However, it does, at least for a time, serve an adaptive and/or defensive purpose in the individual's life.

Substance abuse is merely a symptom of other problems, and it is always associated with other identifiable symptoms. When the only goal of the proffered treatment is abstinence, have we really done anything significant to make the patient's life better? All that was accomplished in a great many instances is that we have robbed the individual of his or her only means of adapting to or coping with an adverse condition. Maybe all we have accomplished is to create individuals who belong to a class of "walking wounded." Our big accomplishment was merely to reduce the list of symptoms by one.

There must be a better way to deal with an individual's psychological dependence upon alcohol and/or other drugs. I believe there is a better way. I will outline a method of treating psychological

dependence upon alcohol and other drugs that I believe holds much
more promise in comparison to traditional twelve-step treatment.

References

Chapter Ten

Alcoholics Anonymous. (2001). *The Story of How More than One hundred Men Have Recovered from Alcoholism. Fourth edition.* (p. 59) New York, NY: Alcoholics Anonymous World Services, Inc.

American Psychiatric Association. (1994). *Diagnostic and Statistical Manual of Mental Disorders, Fourth Edition.* (p. 181).American Psychiatric Association. Washington, DC.

Jellinek, E. M. (1952). Phases of alcohol addiction. *Quarterly Journal of Studies on Alcohol,* **13(4)**, 673–684.

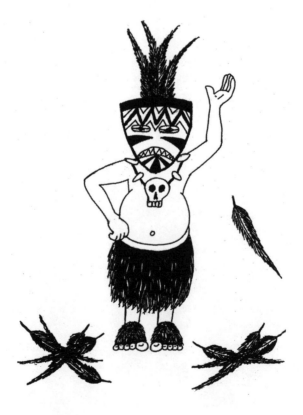

Chapter Eleven

Denial: The Scylla and Charybdis
of Twelve-step Treatment

More than a few research efforts have pointed out some painfully obvious facts regarding how our nation has dealt with substance use disorders. For example, McLellan et al. (1992) concluded that standard detoxification and "twenty-eight day programs" are insufficient to deal with the long-term issues associated with substance abuse and dependence. These conclusions supported the earlier findings of Miller and Hester (1986), which indicated that traditional treatment programs were very expensive, "despite clear evidence that they offer no advantage in overall effectiveness" (p. 163).

In 1990, the Institute of Medicine commissioned a National Academy of Sciences committee to make an extensive critical review of the research literature on treatment for alcohol problems (1990b). Their general conclusion was that there existed "a broad range of activities that vary in content, duration, intensity, goals, setting, provider and target population" (p. 86). The committee published their overall conclusions in *Broadening the Base of Treatment of Alcohol Problems* (1990a). It was stated therein that:

1. There is no single treatment approach that is effective for all persons with alcohol problems.
2. The provision of appropriate, specific treatment modalities can substantially improve outcomes.

3. Brief interventions can be quite effective compared with no treatment, and they can be quite cost effective compared with more intensive treatment.
4. Treatment of other life problems related to drinking can improve outcomes in persons with alcohol problems.
5. Therapist characteristics are partial determinants of outcome.
6. Outcomes are determined in part by treatment process factors, post-treatment adjustment factors, the characteristics of individuals seeking treatment, the characteristics of their problems, and the interactions among these factors.
7. People treated for alcohol problems achieve a continuum of outcomes with respect to drinking behavior and alcohol problems and follow different course of outcome.
8. Those who significantly reduce their level of alcohol consumption or who become totally abstinent usually enjoy improvement in other life areas, particularly as the period of reduced consumption becomes more extended. (pp. 147–148)

The Institute of Medicine ultimately concluded, "Chemical dependency is the treatment with the highest revenues, probably the second largest number of clients, and the smallest scientific basis for assessing its effectiveness" (IOM, 1990a, p. 18).

Do these conclusions sound familiar? They should, because they echo much of what has been stated thus far. Our traditional means of treating substance use disorders is very costly, and it has proven to be ineffective.

Yet, we persist! Despite having an abundant amount of evidence indicating that the way we understand substance abuse problems and the way our nation has attempted to treat substance use disorders has been misguided and ineffective, nothing has changed. As a nation we are in deep *denial* of what must be done to treat substance use disorders effectively, successfully, and affordably.

There it is—the term "denial." *What is denial and why is it important with regard to both our understanding of substance use disorders and how we might go about treating these disorders?* According to *Webster's II New Revised Dictionary* (1984), denial means, "1. the refusal to acknowledge the truth of a statement, or 2. a repudiation: disavowal."

As a nation, we have certainly refused to acknowledge that our common understanding of alcoholism and drug dependency is without factual support. Additionally, despite an ever-increasing amount of evidence clearly indicating that our treatment efforts are both costly and ineffective, we refuse to abandon what has been done for the last two hundred years in favor of trying more promising treatment approaches.

Denial would also accurately describe the state of our existing chemical dependency treatment industry. Those who support the status quo refuse to acknowledge that the disease concept cannot be supported by the truth as evidenced through objective research. The industry has certainly attempted to disavow any evidence lending support to the premise that substance abuse and substance dependency are a symptom of abnormal psychological conditions rather than the result of some ill-defined disease.

So, we have a nation in denial of the truth regarding substance use disorders and the treatment thereof. We also have an entire industry that purports to be dedicated to the treatment of substance use disorders but wants to deny that the treatment is misguided, costly, and wholly ineffective.

Some service providers who treat both substance use and mental health problems understand the term "denial" in a different context. Denial is generally used to identify a phenomenon that is observed when offering treatment services to any patient. Whether patients suffer from a substance use disorder or from a mental health diagnosis, denial is an almost universal initial response to treatment. Denial occurs when the therapist begins to approach a direct discussion of any patient's most apparent and serious problem(s).

In a typical therapeutic scenario, when the therapist initially begins to directly discuss or explore a patient's most glaring problem(s), such as substance use, the affinity to depressive responses, anger, etc., the therapist observes that the patient becomes more anxious or angry, or exhibits an apparent defensive posture. Generally, patients will either overtly or covertly attempt to avoid direct discussions of their problems during the early stages of treatment. Patients may actually deny that they have ever experienced such problems. Any patient is likely to make excuses or blame other persons or circumstances for his or her difficulty and pain. This kind of response from a patient is called denial.

Denial, in a psychological context, is actually a term describing a condition wherein an individual employs one or more psychological defense mechanisms. Without going into a detailed psychoanalytic explanation of defense mechanisms, it is sufficient to simply understand that defense mechanisms serve as a means to psychologically protect an individual. An individual will employ these mechanisms when faced or confronted with information, events, and/or circumstances that threaten the individual's images and perceptions of who he or she is and how the patient fits into the world, or when the individual perceives that there exists a threat to his or her psychological and/or physical well-being. An individual will rely on psychological defenses when his or her sense of balance or normalcy is challenged.

Defense mechanisms are responses that occur in an autonomic manner. In most instances, patients who respond in a defensive manner by exhibiting any number of defense mechanisms do so without conscious awareness of their responses.

All individuals employ defense mechanisms. It is extremely important for any treatment provider to understand that defense mechanisms are behaviors serving an adaptive and protective function for the individual patient. Defense mechanisms allow the patient to defend his or her most intimately held perceptions and images, at least temporarily, until new awareness and understanding can be developed. Defense mechanisms protect the individual's psychological integrity by providing a sort of safety zone wherein the additional skills or insight needed to allow the individual to alter perceptions and internal images to be more congruent with objective reality can be acquired.

All human beings exhibit a denial of reality at times. It is an innate response. When our individual perceptions and beliefs are threatened or challenged, we are all capable of lapsing into denial. Denial is a perfectly natural and normal phenomenon. Being able to rely on the emergence of our natural defenses is essential to the preservation of our overall psychological well-being.

Even though all individuals are likely to rely on defense mechanisms during encounters with various challenging events and circumstances, most individuals also have the capacity to gradually incorporate these events and/or circumstances into their lives in a manner consistent with objective reality. Most individuals develop the capacity to adjust to the challenges of daily living.

However, there are times when an individual can hold on to a defense so stubbornly that it interferes with the ability to acquire new information, knowledge, and skills. Frequently, individuals who become overly reliant upon their respective defenses are people who have, for one reason or another, never obtained the skills needed to reconcile the dissonance experienced when their beliefs and perceptions do not correspond to objective reality. Therapists are then called upon to assist in the facilitation of a realistic adjustment to the events and/or circumstances initiating the defensive posturing.

Denial is considered a primitive response exhibited when an individual feels threatened. Primitive, in this context, means that it is a defensive posture characteristically observed in children or in individuals whose emotional, social, and/or intellectual development has been delayed, arrested, or disrupted. Denial is an immature response to a threatening event or set of circumstances. This does not mean that normal adults never exhibit this kind of defensive posturing.

To provide you with a simple example of how a child might engage in denial, imagine that you walk into your kitchen after having heard the clattering of cupboard or refrigerator doors, knowing that the only other living creature in your home is your three-year-old daughter, Wendy. When you enter the kitchen, you find Wendy's face and hands are completely covered with chocolate frosting. You then confront Wendy by saying, "Wendy, did you eat some of that chocolate cake that I baked for your brother's birthday? Didn't I tell you to leave it alone?" Of course, like most three-year-old children who might perceive that they've done something that might get them into trouble, Wendy responds by stating, "No, Mommy, I didn't do it." You question her, "Well then, how did your face get covered in chocolate?" With a straight face and with a sincere childlike expression, Wendy states, "Buddy ate the cake and then he licked my face all over." You look out the kitchen window and Buddy, the family's cocker spaniel, is sleeping underneath the tree in the backyard, and he is not covered in chocolate frosting.

Now, Wendy knows she ate the cake. Wendy also knows that she wasn't supposed to get into the cake until that evening when the family was going to celebrate her brother's birthday. Wendy fears the consequences of her behavior. Wendy feels threatened that she might be punished for giving in to her impulse. Wendy might even be fearful that if she admits to her behavior that her mother will think she is a bad girl. So, Wendy denies that she ate the cake, and she blames the dog for the missing cake and her chocolate-covered face. It seemed believable to Wendy! It explained everything as far as she was concerned. According to Wendy's immature thinking, her story kept her safe.

Is this realistically any different from how an adult substance abuser might respond when questioned about substance use? Those of you who have spent any time at all in working with substance abusers, or anyone who has lived with one, will easily recognize that the substance abuser frequently denies the use of substances in a manner not all that dissimilar to Wendy's denial of her actions. The substance abuser will often deny using or the extent of his or her substance use, or will manufacture some excuse for his or her use.

Why do adults or even adolescents engage in such transparent lies? There are three reasonable answers to such a question. First, the individual substance abuser is unready or unwilling to face the consequences of the behavior. Second, the individual has not developed the capacity to comprehend or understand how or why the behavior is inappropriate and/or destructive. Third, by admitting to the problem, the individual has to accept that something is wrong, thereby facing the possibility that that he or she is in some way broken or defective in comparison to other "normal" people.

Individuals who suffer from substance use disorders almost universally present in treatment in a state of denial. The degree to which an individual entering treatment may exhibit denial, of course, varies from mild to extreme. At times, the substance abuser can be solidly anchored in denial of problems. This stubborn stance does present a very real and persistent obstacle in any therapeutic effort. As such, assisting the individual patient in overcoming denial is most frequently the very first challenge that must be faced by a therapist when offering treatment to the substance-abusing patient.

Do substance-abusing patients present with a more serious and persistent denial as compared to individuals who might suffer from any other mental illness? The answer to that question is definitely no! Denial is denial. It is the same problem for the individual who suffers from depression, anxiety, or any other problem, as it is for the substance-abusing patient. It is purely an indication that an individual is employing one or more natural defenses. Contrary to popular notions, denial is no more or less of a problem for individuals who abuse mood-altering substances than it is for any other individual who might present for treatment of any other mental health diagnosis.

Denial is, nonetheless, a problem that must be addressed if there is to be any hope of assisting the patient in overcoming any problem. When it comes to treating any mental problem, it is impossible for a patient to make much progress if he or she is unwilling or unable to consider the possibility that there exists a condition requiring correction.

Is denial a difficult problem to overcome? I personally would never say that it is easy for patients to overcome denial. As with any human problem, change never comes easily. On the other hand, if a therapist cannot find appropriate and constructive means of addressing denial with the patient, the therapist is not likely to be of much assistance to any patient regardless of the patient's problem. The plain truth is that denial is a therapeutic concern when dealing with any patient's problems. It's the degree of the patient's denial that determines how big a problem it is when addressing it in therapy.

It must be emphasized that if a therapist sincerely wishes to assist in addressing the patient's overall problem, regardless of whether the patient suffers from a substance abuse disorder or not, the efforts expended to address denial must be appropriate within the context of the patient's problem; undertaken with an understanding and appreciation as to what adaptive and protective function the defense mechanisms are performing; and appreciative of how the patient can be damaged if the patient is suddenly and systematically robbed of the ability to utilize natural and autonomic psychological defenses.

In Chapter One, I offered a definition of alcoholism discovered on the NCADD Web site (2005). Part of that definition stated: "It [alcoholism] is characterized by continuous or periodic: impaired control over drinking, preoccupation with the drug alcohol, use of alcohol despite adverse consequences, and *distortions in thinking, most notably denial*" (emphasis added). According to this definition, alcoholism is characterized by denial. In other words, denial is considered to be a major symptom of alcoholism, and it is explained to be a distortion of the thinking processes exhibited by the alcoholic.

Since the disturbance in thinking, denial, is considered to be a hallmark symptom of alcoholism, then the treatment of alcoholism should specifically target denial; this pervasive distortion of the alcoholic's thought processes is a problem that must be corrected in order for the alcoholic can begin to recover. Well, the good news is that all traditional (meaning twelve-step) treatment models do specifically address denial as a major part of the treatment protocol. The bad news is, for the most part, this is all traditional twelve-step treatment programs do! The really bad news is, because traditional wisdom defines denial as merely a disturbance of thought symptomatic of the disease of alcoholism, the traditional approach to correcting this so-called symptom is misguided and often exceedingly damaging to the patient.

If you will recall the descriptions from individuals who endured traditional twelve-step treatment in Chapter Five, nearly all of the therapeutic actions described were attempts to rid the patient of denial as defined within twelve-step ideology. It might be beneficial for the reader to review the examples provided in that chapter, or to read other first hand accounts of what individuals have experienced in traditional twelve-step treatment programs.

Twelve-step treatment really only accomplishes one singular goal. That goal is to indoctrinate the individual patient into lifelong participation in a twelve-step recovery program, such as Alcoholics Anonymous. This indoctrination can only be accomplished when the alcoholic/addict overcomes the *distortions in thinking* preventing the acceptance that he or she suffers from a disease controllable only by lifelong participation in a twelve-step recovery program.

Let us once again examine what is accomplished in traditional twelve-step treatment.

As previously outlined, twelve-step treatment programs merely attempt to move the substance-abusing patient through the first four steps of the Twelve Steps of Alcoholics Anonymous (2001). These steps are as follows:

1. We admitted that we are powerless over alcohol—that our lives had become unmanageable.
2. Came to believe that a power greater than ourselves could restore us to sanity.
3. Made a decision to turn our will and our lives over to the care of God as we understood him.
4. Made a searching and fearless moral inventory of ourselves.

I have already broken down these steps to expose what is really accomplished when a patient comes to believe in the "inherent truth" brought to light in the process of moving through these steps. These steps are merely an attempt to persuade the patient to think of himself or herself in the following manner: 1) the patient is powerless and cannot manage his or her life; 2) the patient is insane and can only become sane again by accepting the help of a greater power; 3) the patient becomes willing to abandon any notion of self-determination or free-will by turning his or her life over to God (not necessarily the biblical God) who can only be found in a twelve-step recovery program; 4) the patient must acknowledge that he or she is composed of a whole list of undesirable characteristics which render the patient as being no good.

When the patient in the twelve-step treatment program successfully completes these four steps, according to the judgment of a non-professional alcohol and drug counselor, it is assumed that the patient has overcome denial to a sufficient extent that the patient is now ready to embark on the road to recovery. That is, the patient no longer suffers from distortions of thinking that might lead the patient to believe that he or she: 1) has some power to control and manage, at least, some facets of his or her life; 2) is sane enough to continue to live independently without handing total control of his or her life to some outside authority; 3) has some ability to make decisions and choices about what his or her life should be in the present or in the future; 4) does possess some good and redeemable personal characteristics.

Now, after having been purged of the distortions of thinking as outlined above, the patient is fully prepared to enter into lifelong membership in a twelve-step recovery program, such as Alcoholics Anonymous, wherein the patient will be constantly reminded that he or she must never again fall prey to these distortions of thinking. Should the patient ever entertain any notion that he or she is in any way normal or like other sane, powerful, good people who have the ability to make decisions as to how their lives are and should be, the patient will most assuredly end up drunk or dead.

For the life of me, I have never been able to understand how anyone, let alone any person trained in any of the healing professions, could believe that treating a person in this manner is a good idea. This isn't treatment. This is just brainwashing! When a patient is taught to consider himself or herself to be insane, powerless, totally incapable of self-determination, and just no good, what is left? Can there be any question in anyone's mind as to why the most probable outcome to twelve-step treatment is relapse?

However, when you consider that twelve-step treatment is entirely dedicated to indoctrination into twelve-step recovery efforts, it makes sense that it might be necessary to render patients deplete of their normal and natural defenses in order to insure the individual's entry into such a recovery effort. Essentially, when stripped of their defenses, individuals become vulnerable enough to believe that if they don't follow the suggestions of their trusted twelve-step counselors or mentors, they'll either end up drunk or dead.

Stanton Peele (1989) and Charles Bufe (1998) both have referred to how traditional treatment programs and twelve-step recovery groups have utilized the twelve-step view of denial in ways that create catch-22 scenarios for those who become involved in treatment and recovery efforts. Bufe said:

Denial is a catch-22 concept, and as such is essentially useless except as a bludgeon in the indoctrination process—if you admit that you're an alcoholic, you're an alcoholic; and if you deny that you're an alcoholic, you're in denial, which is evidence that you're an alcoholic. Either way, as with denials of witchcraft in the Middle Ages, you lose. (1998)

Peele stated:

Modern treatment philosophy insists that denial is a keystone of alcoholism and must be attacked before recovery can occur. Yet we have seen that people from different cultural backgrounds and with varied personal experiences may view drinking and alcoholism very differently. The picture of different views of alcoholism does not indicate that those who don't accept that they have a "disease" should be attacked and converted to a particular treatments point of view. Nonetheless, the standard approach in the alcoholism movement is to bombard problem drinkers with the disease message until their previous beliefs are exorcised and, thus purified, they can join the movement. (1989)

NCADD and others who ascribe to twelve-step ideology have created a unique and special definition when it comes to their use of the term *denial*. It is apparent that their conceptualization of denial is terribly misguided. Such a unique definition might be justified if it could be demonstrated that the understanding of denial, as defined, could be used to the benefit of individuals who suffer from substance use disorders. Unfortunately, this "special" definition and treatment of the term denial represents the introduction of yet another mythical concept intended to serve as a misdirection to persuade vulnerable individuals to accept the mystical twelve-step approach to treatment and recovery.

Denial is not simply "distortions in thinking." Denial is not limited to alcoholics or addicts. People who are considered to be perfectly normal, sane, and good exhibit denial from time to time. While it is certainly true that individuals in denial do appear to exhibit distortions of thinking related to specific aspects of their lives or to specific behaviors; more often than not, these individuals can also handle many facets of their respective lives in a perfectly normal and acceptable manner.

Remember, denial may represent a number of psychological defense mechanisms that serve a protective and adaptive function for any individual—alcoholics and addicts included. To obliterate or completely strip an individual of the ability to activate any of the defense mechanisms accomplishes nothing except to render the individual exceedingly vulnerable to outside influences. Simply, the individual becomes psychologically defenseless. Any effort directed toward complete and total neutralization of an individual's psychological defenses cannot be considered therapeutic, ethical, or even advisable. But, this is exactly what twelve-step treatment attempts to accomplish—the elimination of denial as it is defined by twelve-step ideology.

Is there a better way to deal with denial? Any well-trained and competent therapist can appropriately and constructively deal with patient denial in the course of assisting the patient in overcoming substance use, depression, anxiety, or any other problem presenting itself in therapy. Real therapists deal with denial on a daily basis. Furthermore, they do so in a manner that does not debilitate their patients!

Denial, in many patients, is marked by a sense of confusion. That is, most patients, even those who suffer substance use disorders, do on some level understand that something is wrong. They know that, for some reason, life just isn't working out for them in some aspect when they compare their perceptions of the lives of others to their own. These patients have not yet developed the ability or the willingness to isolate the reasons for their inappropriate and destructive behavior. They certainly have not yet developed the ability to offer the therapist or the counselor accurate verbal explanations as to what is wrong with them. They just know that their life isn't working and they cannot get a handle on just why this is so.

This is what denial looks like in most patients. For many patients, it is not that they are constitutionally unwilling to acknowledge defects in character, genetic defects, or their disease. Individuals exhibit denial when they are truly uncertain as to what is wrong with them, and when they fear what they might have to face. Essentially, denial represents the manifestation and utilization of psychological defenses which are autonomic, natural, and unconscious defenses against feelings of fear and uncertainty.

Should the therapist respond to this confusion and lack of understanding, or insight, by verbally assaulting the patient? Should the therapist respond to the patient by shouting, "Bullshit! You know exactly what's wrong with you. You know why you are here. Just admit it"? Should the therapist go on to tell the patient that they are certain that the patient suffers from some inherent disease from which there is no absolute recovery? Should the therapist then explain to the patient that he or she never was and never will be like other "normal people"?

I could certainly understand that a patient who is the recipient of such an onslaught of confrontation on the part of any counselor or therapist might not be willing to return for continuing therapy or treatment. Nevertheless, a large percentage of those admitted into twelve-step treatment programs in our nation are coerced into participation by the courts, their employers, or their families. These patients have little choice as to whether or not they might wish to endure this type of treatment. They either endure this abuse in the name of treatment, or they risk being jailed or losing their profession or family. This is the reality of treatment for addictions in this nation.

How can denial, as it is properly defined, be addressed in a therapeutic manner so as to avoid robbing patients of their innate psychological defenses thereby rendering them psychologically defenseless? There are probably many answers to this question. For the moment, let's just say that any effort on the part of a therapist to address denial should be undertaken by utilizing an approach that allows the therapist to be understanding, patient yet persistent, and fully appreciative of what the patients' defensive posturing is accomplishing.

I believe that the effective and therapeutic treatment of denial must take the form of a process, not a singular intervention. The therapist must approach the patient's defensive posturing with an understanding that it may take some time for the patient to gradually abandon currently held perceptions and images for perceptions and images more congruent to objective reality. The therapist must appreciate that the patient's reliance upon a given defense is predicated on his or her immediate inability to face the events and circumstances causing the patient to experience overwhelming and debilitating fear and uncertainty. Most importantly, the therapist must be able to recognize which defenses the patient is exhibiting and which functions those defenses are performing.

The first step in effectively addressing denial is to completely abandon the conceptualization of denial as it has been offered by proponents of twelve-step ideology. Twelve-step ideology promotes the notion that the term denial is descriptive of distortions of thinking which are expressly symptomatic of and consequential to the disease of alcoholism. Actually, what occurs when an individual enters a state of denial is that the person's innate and largely unconscious natural defenses have emerged as a means of protecting the individual from overwhelming feelings of fear and uncertainty. These distortions of thinking may actually represent a whole list of distinct and separate psychological defenses that can be exhibited by an addicted person, or for that matter, any person. Even normal individuals employ defense mechanisms.

Let us take a look at what most therapists recognize in terms of psychological defense mechanisms. These are listed and defined in abnormal psychology textbooks such as *Understanding Abnormal Behavior* (Sue, Sue, and Sue, 1990) as follows:

1. Repression—the blocking of forbidden or dangerous desires and thoughts to keep them from entering into consciousness.
2. Reaction Formation—dangerous impulses or thoughts are repressed and then converted to their opposites.

3. Projection – people rid themselves of threatening thoughts or desires by attributing them to others.
4. Rationalization—a person provides well-thought-out and socially acceptable reasons for certain behaviors, but these reasons do not happen to be the real ones.
5. Displacement—directing an emotion such as hostility or anxiety toward a substitute target (sometimes referred to as scapegoating).
6. Undoing—a symbolic attempt to right a wrong or negate some disapproved thought, impulse, or act.
7. Regression—retreating to an earlier developmental level that demands less mature responses and aspirations.

These are the defense mechanisms most therapists recognize. Therapists employ established therapeutic techniques to systematically address these defenses during the course of therapy if they, indeed, present obstacles to the patient's progress.

It is easy to see why these defenses can be seen, on the surface, as being distortions of thinking. A person engaging in any of theses defenses appears to be suffering from cognitive distortions. However, these defenses are not engaged on a conscious level, they occur autonomically. More importantly, these defenses emerge as a means of defending an individual from feelings of uncertainty and fear until a more appropriate response can be formulated on a conscious level. And, finally, an individual does not have to be mentally ill or substance-dependent to exhibit these defenses.

When a competent therapist says that a patient is in denial, what the therapist is really referring to is that the patient is exhibiting any one of a combination of any of these defense mechanisms. A well-qualified therapist recognizes that he or she is observing the manifestation of these defenses simply because the patient is, at that point in time, unable to acknowledge what he or she is actually experiencing because such a realization would be overwhelming to the patient. Essentially, what this means is that the patient is either incapable or unwilling to acknowledge the reality of the behavior because the individual fears what acceptance of that reality will mean, or the patient simply does not know how to effectively and appropriately respond to that reality.

Bludgeoning and badgering a patient until the individual quits using psychological defenses does not render the reality of what a patient might need to accept as any less overwhelming. As we have seen, the twelve-step approach to dealing with denial leaves the patient psychologically vulnerable and overwhelmed because the patient is forced and coerced into acknowledging and accepting a reality for which the patient is ill prepared to accommodate. The reason that the patient is in denial is because the patient fears what must be faced. The patient has not developed a means of incorporating or converting what is experienced into something that can readily fit into existing perceptions and beliefs as to what objective reality is. If what the patient is observing is a reality which is inconsistent with internal images and perceptions, that means either the patient must question what is observed or experienced, or the patient must assume that his or her personal and unique vision of objective reality is inaccurate or untrue. Ask yourself which of these two possible responses you believe you would choose if you were to be confronted with an event or set of circumstances for which you were unprepared to face upon demand.

Previously, I indicated that I believe that there is a better way to deal with denial.

I will now describe the primary process that I have utilized with patients that does not require them to abandon their psychological defenses until they have developed the ability to do so without experiencing overwhelming fear and uncertainty.

In Chapter Seven, I outlined the importance of creating an operational definition of a patient's problem. This process of creating an operational definition is accomplished by having the therapist, in collaboration with the patient, compile as complete and thorough a history of the patient's physical, psychological, social, and even spiritual development as possible. When this is accomplished, as was outlined, the therapist then has a contextual landscape from which he or she can identify specific events, experiences, and circumstances that may have contributed to the problems the patient is experiencing.

This is an extremely important process in terms of facilitating the therapist's ability to accurately identify specific problems and thereby devise treatment approaches that are likely to be relevant to the patient's life experiences and the patient's way of relating to world. It is also an important process for the patient. From the patient's perspective, it allows the patient the opportunity to also review his or her life experiences. When a patient is given this opportunity, he or she is encouraged to view life experiences in more objective terms. Essentially, participation in this cooperative exploration of the personal life history gives the patient an opportunity to develop insight and understanding as to how and why there are currently problems which must be faced. This is a major step in overcoming denial.

By the time a competent therapist arrives at a point in the evaluation process wherein the therapist can identify specific diagnoses of a patient's problems and devise relevant treatment plans for the patient, the patient has gained significant insight and understanding of the problem(s) as well. It may not always be that a patient will agree with exactly what a therapist offers as a diagnosis or a treatment plan. In most instances, however, the patient may be ready to consider what the therapist offers as an explanation of the problem, and that patient may be much more willing to approach a problem in a manner suggested by the therapist.

In more than twenty years of experience in offering treatment for substance use problems and other mental health issues, I can honestly tell you that I can count on my fingers the number of patients who have overtly rejected my assessment of their problems, or who have stated strong objections to my suggestions as a means to help them overcome their respective problems. Most often by that point in the therapeutic process, patients have gained sufficient insight into and understanding of their problems to risk trying some things not previously considered as realistic alternatives. They are beginning to realize that they are experiencing some identifiable problems. They are frequently also ready to consider the possibility that there might be some realistic way to correct these problems as well. Essentially, by assisting patients to create a literal road map as to how and why they have come to create the life they are now experiencing, patients might not find the fear and uncertainty as to what they are experiencing to be quite so overwhelming.

If all that I described comes to pass, does that mean that the patient's denial has been fully addressed? In some instances, the answer to this question is yes. It is very possible that for some patients, substance-abusing patients included, simply helping them develop some basic understanding and insight into the how and why they have developed the problems they are experiencing is all that must be done to sufficiently address their state of denial. More often than not, however, patients will continue to rely on their defense mechanisms when they feel that they are being psychologically threatened in some way.

Denial is a manifest expression indicating that a patient is employing one or more innate and natural defense mechanisms. Goals of therapy should never be created with the intention of completely neutralizing any patient's utilization of innate defenses. Defense mechanisms contributing to denial should only be addressed or confronted when they present as significant obstacles to the patient's ability to develop new insight, understanding, and skills to assist in the process of incorporating events, experiences, thoughts, and emotions into the patient's perceptions of objective reality. Even then, denial should only be addressed to the extent that it no longer prohibits the patient from continuing to make progress in treatment.

Over the years, it has been my practice to create a provision included within the written treatment plan created for any patient. It states that the patient has read the treatment plan; is in agreement with the goals and objectives stated within the treatment plan; and is willing to abide by the treatment plan. Actually, in many states, there are rules and regulations requiring therapists to include such provisions in treatment plans.

When a patient willingly signs this provision, this serves as an indication that the patient's denial has been addressed to the extent that it is unlikely that this denial will continue to represent a significant obstacle prohibiting the patient from making progress in a therapeutic effort. In essence, the patient's willingness to sign this provision offers an acknowledgement of an identifiable problem. It also offers the acknowledgement that there may be another means of addressing this problem besides that which has already been tried. When I see a patient willing to take these actions, I can't really state that his or her denial is truly an obstacle to treatment! Yes, defense mechanisms may continue to appear from time to time throughout the treatment effort. The defenses may even slow the patient's progress for a time. However, these can be addressed if and when it is appropriate to do so. What most therapists understand is that individuals, all individuals, need to be able to make use of their defenses at times. Utilizing a defense does not always indicate resistance to the therapeutic effort, nor is it an indication of a problem. It may just mean that the patient has touched upon something that he or she doesn't immediately know how to face. This is what treatment is—helping patients to face and deal with problems in more constructive and effective ways!

What happens when a therapist offers a diagnosis of the patient's problem and lays out a plan of action to correct those problems, and because of denial, the patient rejects what the therapist is offering? The answer to that question is simple: terminate the therapeutic effort!

If a patient completely rejects the diagnosis, and cannot or will not go along with the treatment plan, the therapist has little choice but to honor the patient's decision. Remember our discussion of informed consent?

Therapists and counselors must always be cognizant that patients can always, at any time that they might choose, exercise freedom of choice. Even if their reason for doing so is that they are in denial. This holds true even for patients who are court mandated to seek treatment. No court in our nation has the legal authority to make any individual seek specific treatment or to submit to the treatment of any specific treatment provider. Even those individuals who are judged to be mentally incompetent by a legal authority can still refuse treatment.

When patients refuse treatment, the therapist should make an effort to explain the possible consequences of such a refusal. This should be approached with the appreciation that the patient is acting within his or her right to exercise free will. The therapist may also offer to arrange referral to another provider if the patient is willing to accept a referral.

What a therapist should never do is aggressively confront the patient by insisting that the patient is in denial and then proceed to emotionally bludgeon the patient until he or she relents and reluctantly agrees to whatever is asked. All this accomplishes is to place the patient between Scylla and Charybdis. From this position, all the patient can do is make a choice between two evils. As we have seen from historical perspective and as evidenced by the utter failure of twelve-step treatment, it is unlikely that this will serve to accomplish anything positive to help the patient to overcome substance use or any other problem.

Yes, substance abusers do rely on their defense mechanisms. So do individuals who do not abuse substances. I do, and so do you. We all deny our reality at times. Does that mean we all suffer from a disease characterized by distorted thinking? I guess we can say that we all suffer from the disease of living. There are times when I really need to deny the reality of what I observe, even if it's just for a little while. As therapists, we need to acknowledge that our patients have that right as well. We don't need to rob them of that in order to be helpful.

References

Chapter Eleven

Alcoholics Anonymous. (2001). *The Story of How More than One Hundred Men Have Recovered from Alcoholism. Fourth Edition.* New York, NY: Works Publishing Company, Inc.

Bufe, C. (1998). AA's Impact on Society. *Alcoholics Anonymous: Cult or Cure.* 2nd Edition, revised. San Francisco, CA: See Sharp Press.

Gil, M. (1982). *Analysis of transference.* Vol. 1, Psychological Issues, 353. New York, NY: International Universities Press.

Institute of Medicine. (1990a). *Broadening the base of treatment for alcohol problems.* Washington, DC: National Academy Press.

Institute of Medicine. (1990b). *Treating drug problems (Vol. 1).* Washington, DC: National Academy Press.

Miller, W. R., and Hester, R. K. (1986). The effectiveness of alcoholism treatment: What research reveals. W. R. Miller and N. Heather (Eds.), *Treating Addictive Behaviors: Process of Change* (pp. 121–172). New York, NY: Plenum.

National Council on Alcoholism and Drug Dependence. (2005). Definition of alcoholism. Web site: http://www.ncadd.org/facts/defalc.html.

Peele, S. (1989). *Diseasing of America: How We Allowed Recovery Zealots and the Treatment Industry To Convince We Are Out Of Control.* (p. 79) New York, NY: Lexington Books.

Sue, D., Sue, D, and Sue, G. (1990). *Understanding Abnormal Behavior.* 3rd Edition (pp. 42–43). Boston, MA: Houghton Mifflin Company.

Webster's II New Riverside Dictionary. (1984). (p. 190). Boston, MA: Houghton Mifflin Company

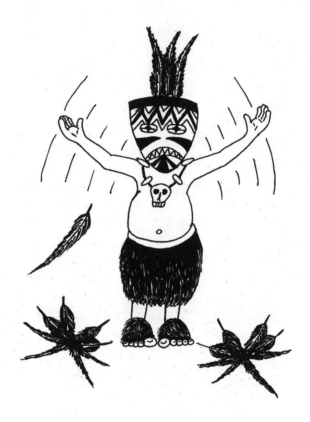

Chapter 12

Laying a Foundation for Effective Treatment

Up to this point we have covered a lot of ground regarding our discussion of addiction and what has historically been done in attempts to treat these problems. It is time to move past all of this in an effort to outline a more promising means of addressing substance use disorders.

Before we jump right into descriptions of the specific treatment strategies that I have found to be truly effective, I must take just a little time to discuss some practical matters that must be considered in relation to the provision of treatment services. This would include such considerations as what might be appropriate in terms of treatment levels or settings, in addition to a number of other important matters that need to be given some attention in order to make our treatment efforts effective in terms of positive outcomes and cost efficiency. In other words, I need to describe what kind of foundation needs to be laid to facilitate an effective treatment effort.

Some important considerations that should be given attention in laying foundation for effective treatment include the following: What kind of facility is needed to provide treatment with a reasonable chance for success? What kind of treatment providers need to be employed? How much treatment do individuals really need? How long should that treatment take in order to be successful? These are some important questions that really need to be addressed before we begin to specifically describe what type of interventions will be implemented.

Treatment Setting. The overwhelming majority of formal treatment programs created within the last forty years can be described as short-term inpatient treatment efforts using the traditional twelve-step model. Most of these programs have required patients to be hospitalized for twenty-eight days, more or less. In recent years, programs offering twelve-step treatment were offered giving patients choices between outpatient and intensive outpatient, or day treatment settings. The only real difference between traditional inpatient treatment and these alternative program settings is that the latter do not require the patients to be hospitalized or otherwise sequestered from their families and the public. It must be emphasized that the actual treatment provided within all of these settings is the same. It remains that more than 90 percent of all of these programs offer twelve-step treatment and little else.

Outpatient, intensive outpatient, and day treatment programs were created in response to the health-care industry's desire to limit the costs of addictions treatment, not to any industry demand for alternative types of treatments.

For our purposes, we will look at traditional twenty-eight-day inpatient treatment as the standard upon which all treatment efforts are compared. We have already described what treatment in these programs look like. We have also discussed what the goals of this treatment are intend to accomplish and how effective this approach has been in assisting patients overcome substance use problems. As much as possible, I will attempt to dispense with a rehashing of material we have already discussed at length.

Traditional twenty-eight-day treatment programs require that patients remain within the treatment facility twenty-four hours a day for the duration. Patients may be transported to twelve-step meetings outside the facility from time to time, and patients may, in some instances, be allowed short leaves of absence. Excursions outside the treatment facility are the exception, not the rule. Overall, patients in most inpatient programs are prohibited from leaving the treatment facility until they are discharged.

Why do substance-abusing patients need to be placed in a hospital-like setting for twenty-eight days? During my research, I found no cogent explanation as to why it might be important to sequester a substance-abusing patient. Placing patients in a hospital setting for a period of any where from three to fourteen days might be advisable during withdrawal. However, detoxification of substance-using patients has generally been separate from traditional treatment for addictions. I suspect that the practice of removing a substance-abusing patient from the home environment during treatment is based more on tradition than upon any demonstrated benefit. That is, it is done this way because this has been the practice historically.

As has already been outlined, in the early 1900s, alcoholics and drug addicts were sometimes placed in psychiatric hospitals or sanitariums for a period of time (Nace, 1993) to "dry out" or "kick the habit." According to numerous accounts, this practice had no lasting impact upon the alcoholic's or addict's desire to continue using. The overwhelming majority of these individuals returned to the use of alcohol and/or drugs shortly after they were released.

Later, when AA's Dr. Bob began to offer treatment for alcoholism (Alcoholics Anonymous World Services, 1980), this tradition of sequestering alcoholics was perpetuated. The hospitalization of patients for the purpose of providing treatment for alcoholism and other addictions has carried into modern times because that's what has always been done. If it was a good idea according to Dr. Bob, then it must be right!

Superficially, it might be prudent to remove substance abusing patients from their daily environments to limit access to mood-altering chemicals. By doing so, it can be reasoned that patients are afforded an opportunity to experience a period of chemical free existence while in treatment. Unfortunately, patients do gain access to mood-altering chemicals even while sequestered. Such events have likely been the exception and not the rule. Nonetheless, it has happened with enough regularity that even the most ardent supporters of such practices have to admit that sequestering a patient does not guarantee patients in treatment will remain substance-free.

The most important argument against hospitalization during treatment is that historically it hasn't proven to benefit the patient in any way. Miller and Hester's treatment survey (1986) indicated that hospital (or inpatient) treatment is no better than far less expensive outpatient treatment. Other studies offering comparisons of inpatient versus outpatient treatment effectiveness have supported these observations (Holden, 1987; Nathan and Skinstad, 1987; Mojtabai and Zivin, 2003; Weithmann and Hoffmann, 2005).

So, if it has never been demonstrated that hospitalizing a patient during treatment is effective, why continue such a practice?

In the early 1990s, I was given an opportunity to implement an alcohol and drug treatment program of my own design. In the beginning, all that existed was a grant proposal—a rough idea of what the treatment program was intended to accomplish in terms of outcome along with a brief description of how it was to accomplish desired outcomes. I will describe the implementation of this program as a means to illustrate those practical considerations that must be taken into account prior to the actual delivery of effective and cost-efficient treatment.

The first decision was whether or not the program's treatment services were going to be offered on an inpatient or an outpatient basis. Inpatient treatment offered no real advantages over outpatient efforts in terms of overall effectiveness, and was much less cost-effective, both for the provider and the patient. Additionally, the requirements to license an inpatient treatment program were much more extensive than those to license an outpatient treatment program. The decision was easy: outpatient treatment was the obvious choice.

The next decision concerned how much time patients would need to devote each day to treatment. The proposed program was intended to offer an intensity of treatment comparable to traditional inpatient services. Therefore, patients would have to spend a significant portion of the day involved in the services offered. The program was also designed to allow patients to remain with their families, to work at their jobs, and to remain in their daily environments. To meet these objectives, patients would be required to attend treatment a minimum of ten hours per week. Now, ten hours of treatment may not sound comparable to the services offered in a traditional inpatient program. However, a comparison will be made of the actual services devoted to treatment in a traditional inpatient program to those offered in my program. It will be demonstrated that ten hours of actual treatment activities can closely approximate, and even exceed, that which is provided in most traditional inpatient programs.

Let's examine the daily schedule of services that is offered to patients during their stay at a traditional inpatient program. Outlined below is a schedule for Monday through Friday. Most traditional inpatient programs do not generally require patients to participate in services on weekends or on recognized holidays.

Patient Daily Schedule (Monday – Friday)

7:00–7:55 AM	Wake up and shower time
8:00–8:55 AM	Breakfast
9:00–9:55 AM	Morning lecture
10:00–10:20 AM	Coffee break or free time
10:30–11:45 AM	Twelve-step education
12:00–1:00 PM	Lunch
1:15–2:45 PM	Group therapy
2:45–3:15 PM	Afternoon break
3:20–4:20 PM	Individual therapy
4:20–6:00 PM	Free time
6:00–7:00 PM	Evening meal
7:10–8:30 PM	AA or NA meeting
8:30–10:00 PM	Free time
10:00 PM	Bedtime

This represents a daily schedule which is descriptive of services offered in a traditional inpatient program. Let's look closely at this schedule to determine how much actual treatment an individual patient receives while participating in such a treatment regimen.

First, counselors or other professional treatment personnel would be required to work eight hours per day, Monday through Friday. It is likely that counselors and other professionals would be at the treatment facility from 8:00 AM to 5:00 PM. At all other times, nights, weekends and holidays, the only personnel present would be non-professional individuals who are only required to observe patients and maintain order. A licensed nurse might be required to be present during these times to provide prescribed medication and attend to other health issues. All treatment services offered to patients would have to occur between 8:00 am and 5:00 PM.

Well, as you can see, patients eat their breakfast between 8:00 AM and 8:55 AM. While this is a necessary activity, there's no treatment.

At 9:00 AM, patients are required to attend a morning lecture for approximately an hour. The topic of this morning lecture frequently consists of information related to the "disease" of addiction. The lecture is followed by a twenty to twenty-five minute coffee break.

Then, patients are required to attend one hour and fifteen minutes of twelve-step education. This effort frequently describes each of the Twelve Steps of AA. It may include a discussion as to what patients might expect to experience as they progress through the steps and how they might be expected to benefit.

Lunch! Again, it is necessary but not treatment.

After lunch, it's group therapy time. In previous chapters, we have already detailed what is provided in the name of group therapy: a designated time and place to confront each patient regarding the denial of their "disease." To be fair, some programs may narrowly address other issues relevant to the patients' addictions. Considering this possibility, we will count this time as being spent in actual therapy.

After group therapy, there is the afternoon break followed by an hour allocated for the provision of individual therapy. It is important to note that this does not mean that each patient will be given an hour of individual therapy each day. What this means is that counselors allocate one hour each day to provide individual therapy to one individual. Counselors may have caseloads varying from five to ten patients. If a counselor has a caseload of ten patients, which is about average, during a week the counselors sees five out of ten patients for an individual counseling session. So, an average stay is twenty-eight days or four weeks. This means each patient receives two individual counseling sessions during their entire stay in treatment. This may sound unbelievable. It is, nonetheless, true.

The biweekly individual therapy session is followed by free time and the evening meal.

In the evening, most traditional inpatient programs offer twelve-step support groups. Frequently, AA and NA meetings alternate. Some programs make these mandatory; some do not. These meetings are usually well attended. Patients have little else to do. In addition, some programs allow the outside public to attend, thereby giving patients some opportunity to have contact with individuals who are not patients.

Some programs allow for family counseling on Saturdays; many do not. Additionally, many programs have weekend AA and NA meetings. Beyond these two possible activities, patients are merely housed on the weekends and on holidays.

So, let's add it up. Each day, Monday through Friday, each patient gets one and one half hours of group therapy. Then, each patient might be afforded, at best, one hour of individual therapy each week. This allowance for individual therapy is generous when considering that counselor caseloads are, on average, ten patients. It is more likely that a patient gets one session every other week. Okay, that's one and a half hours of group therapy, times five days, added to the possible one hour of individual therapy per week. That comes to a grand total of eight and a half hours of actual treatment per week. So, in a four week period an individual in inpatient treatment may receive a total of thirty-four hours of actual therapy!

What about the time patients spend in the morning lecture and in twelve-step education? If the morning lectures cover topics and issues relating to the disease concept of addiction, can that be considered actual therapy or treatment? Attempting to teach patients to believe that they suffer from some indefinable disease does not qualify as a therapeutic intervention. Attempting to instruct patients to follow the mystical twelve-step path to overcome their indefinable, mythical disease isn't treatment either!

To sum this up, we can reasonably state that in an average traditional twelve-step, twenty-eight-day inpatient program each patient receives a grand total of thirty-four hours of actually therapy. That's just eight and a half hours per week. The rest is indoctrination into twelve-step ideology.

As can be seen, a proposal to offer a minimum of ten hours of treatment per week would represent more actual therapy than a traditional twenty-eight-day inpatient program would offer. How, you might ask, can this be possible? It is not only possible to accomplish this, but if such an effort is undertaken in a logical and systematic manner, it actually serves a great many more patients per day.

Let's look at how this can be accomplished.

First, all the time and effort that, in a traditional inpatient program, is devoted to nonsensically indoctrinating patients into believing that they suffer from some sort of mythical disease is to be discarded. It is not wrong to inform patients as to the facts regarding addiction. Actually, it is the responsibility of any therapist or treatment program to educate patients. Attempting to convince patients that their addiction is the result of some disease is simply irresponsible and unethical. If time and effort is to be expended educating patients, why not spend that time and effort imparting information that is truthful and beneficial?

Second, convincing individuals who are psychologically dependent upon alcohol or drugs that they can only surmount their problems if they adhere to the teachings of the Alcoholics Anonymous organization is analogous to sending a soldier into combat armed only with a bottle opener. The so-armed soldier might survive a battle, but his survival will have been dependent upon pure chance or other variables not likely to be associated with the bottle opener. The same is true of offering twelve-step methodology to a patient in the guise of treatment for addiction. The patient might surmount the addiction, but recovery will have been 95 percent dependent upon pure chance or other variables not likely associated with the twelve-step path to recovery.

Eliminating the activities traditionally devoted to these two misguided endeavors leaves one and one half hours devoted to group therapy and, perhaps, one hour weekly devoted to individual therapy. Of course, inpatient treatment does offer meals, free time, and a dormitory-style sleeping arrangements. Outpatient programs don't usually offer these latter accoutrements. Well, I don't know about anyone else, but if I'm going to spend more than one thousand dollars per day for meals and personal accommodations, it would certainly be my expectation that I should be able to find better food, more rewarding and fulfilling recreational opportunities, and finer personal sleeping accommodations that can be found in any inpatient treatment facility in this nation. For what most inpatient treatment facilities charge for treatment, one could almost afford to take a thirty-day vacation and take their personal therapist with them!

Now, look at how treatment for addictions can be structured to have a direct and demonstrable positive effect on the patients' disorder, and how these services can be much more cost-effective. But, let's also restrict the number of days devoted to treatment each week a little more, just to make it more challenging. We want to offer our patients, at minimum, ten hours of real, theory-based treatment per week. But, let's do that in four days, not five. Instead of structuring services amounting to two hours of treatment per day, five days a week, we would create a schedule of services requiring our patients to attend treatment for two and a half hours per day for just four days each week. These ten hours would be comprised of a combination of psycho-educational activities, group therapy, and individual therapy directed solely toward assisting patients to overcome their psychological dependence upon alcohol and/or drugs.

A schedule of these services might look something like this:

Morning Schedule of services

9:00–9:55 AM	Pyscho-educational group
10:00–11:30 AM	Group therapy
Individual therapy	Arranged by appointment

Counselors/therapists would provide each patient assigned to them with one hour of individual therapy per week. Individual therapy can be substituted for psycho-educational group for each patient one day per week. Appointments for individual therapy can also be scheduled on Fridays when needed. Family therapy can also be substituted for psycho-educational group as needed.

The example schedule of services as outlined above can also be implemented for afternoon hours such as 1:00 PM to 3:30 PM, or during evening hours from 7:00 PM to 9:30 PM.

A flexible schedule creates a treatment scenario enabling patients to remain in their home environments, with their families, and on the job.

Providing a minimum of ten hours of direct therapy meets the services criteria for intensive outpatient treatment according to most state authorities. Criteria may vary slightly from state to state.

It is entirely possible to create an intensive outpatient treatment program that will provide as much, or even more, direct treatment in comparison to most traditional inpatient treatment facilities.

Facility Requirements. All states in our nation have basic requirements for an alcohol and drug treatment facility or program to be legally licensed. If a treatment program or facility is licensed by state authorities, it must meet state and local building codes, requirements for human occupancy, fire codes, disability access requirements, health and safety standards, and a host of other requirements. Meeting these requirements is part of laying a solid foundation for the provision of treatment.

The requirements to license an inpatient treatment program are much more extensive and expensive than those needed for an intensive outpatient or simple outpatient treatment program. Inpatient treatment programs and facilities must provide patients with meals, sleeping and other personal accommodations, and access to onsite medical care. Intensive outpatient and outpatient treatment programs do not have these housing requirements.

The primary differences between the licensing requirements for intensive outpatient and simple outpatient treatment reside mostly in the amount of services made available to patients. Facilities do not have to differ much between levels of treatment.

Meeting licensing requirements is not an overwhelming task as long as an administrator is willing to abide by the all of the requirements outlined by state licensing authorities. Programs or facilities come under the state's licensing scrutiny only when administrators and program directors attempt to take shortcuts or ignore licensing requirements. These standards are intended to ensure the safety and well being of the patients, which should be very important in the treatment providers' minds as well. Personally,

I have never found it to be that difficult to license even the most humble of treatment facilities.

One of the big advantages of providing treatment on an outpatient basis is that almost any type of building can meet licensing requirements. I have successfully implemented and licensed treatment programs in storefront locations, office and administrative buildings, school buildings, and juvenile group homes. The type of building is not as important as what is provided within that building. All that is required is that a facility has adequate space and rooms to provide private offices for staff, rooms that are large enough to conduct group activities, and secure storage for patient records and other materials that are important to the success of the overall program. If these requirements are met, along with all the other physical requirements, such as fire codes and handicap accessibility, the treatment program is set to go.

Cost Effectiveness. Why does inpatient treatment for addictions cost so much? There are many answers to this question. To avoid a controversial discussion of profit motivations, I'll just state that it costs a great deal more to provide inpatient treatment compared to the provision of the same services in outpatient treatment programs.

When you look at inpatient treatment, there is considerable cost associated with the provision of meals, lodging, access to medical services, maintenance, security, and personnel. Outpatient treatment programs do not have to contend with the high costs associated with the provision of meals and around-the-clock lodging of patients.

While outpatient treatment does share some of the same costs as do inpatient treatment facilities, such as security, maintenance, and so on, these costs are not as high due to the fact that outpatient treatment facilities do not have to operate twenty-four hours a day, 365 days a year.

Outpatient treatment programs do not have as much overhead costs as do inpatient treatment programs. Added to that, if an outpatient program can be structured and administered as simply and directly as possible, the overhead costs of operations drop dramatically. There are huge differences in the overhead cost of a treatment program that must contribute to the support of a large administrative structure in addition to paying program staff and covering operating costs when compared to programs administered by only one or two persons. When a treatment program can operate simply and cost-effectively, considerable savings in terms of cost for services can be passed on to patients.

Addictions treatment programs have historically operated well beyond their income-generating potentials. This, in turn, has caused the cost of treatment services to escalate to the point that most individuals cannot afford treatment for their addiction problems unless they have health insurance to cover the cost of treatment, or if their household incomes are sufficiently low as to qualify the family to receive state and/or federal health-care assistance.

Today, it is not at all unusual for traditional twenty-eight-day inpatient treatment for addictions to cost an individual patient anywhere from fourteen thousand dollars to more than fifty thousand dollars (Roman and Blum, 1997). It has been a long time since I personally have heard of any place wherein a patient could expect to pay less than one thousand dollars per day for inpatient treatment. This is too expensive to be affordable for most individuals and families. The expense of such treatment is amplified even further when it is considered exactly what is offered to patients in the name of treatment. Let's face it: one thousand dollars or more per day for possibly two hours or so of actual treatment is just insane!

What if I contend that a person could receive two and a half hours of actual direct theory-based addictions treatment services for as little as one hundred fifty dollars per day. Could that be possible? It is possible to provide effective treatment services to addicted patients for that low price. I know it is true because I've done it. At that rate, it is even possible for a treatment program to financially support itself and make a small but real profit!

I'll bet you don't believe me. Well, let me prove it to you. Let's create an intensive outpatient treatment program that provides two and a half hours of treatment service per day, four days a week, to each patient.

Okay, our hypothetical treatment program has a staff of four licensed counselors, two education specialists, one program director, and one full-time clerical/support person. Each one of these positions is a salaried position. Annual salaries including fringe benefits are as follows:

Program Director	$ 48,000
Counselors (x 4)	$129,600
Education Specialists (x 2)	$ 52,800
Clerical	$ 18,000
Total personnel cost	$248,400

In a treatment program, your personnel is generally your biggest cost. After all, the program's personnel are also its biggest asset because they generate the program's income. Let us say that personnel costs represent 70 percent of the overall cost of the program, which is realistic if the program design is kept simple. Therefore, a total program budget can be projected as requiring a total of approximately $350,000 to support the program for one year.

Let us say that this program secures a cost-for-service contract with the state. This means that the state will pay a fixed amount of money for every service that is delivered to patients who qualify for state assistance. The typical state's reimbursement rates are as follows:

Group therapy and psycho-educational group	$30 per hour
Individual therapy	$65 per hour
Family therapy	$70 per hour

The program is designed to operate by charging only this rate to all patients regardless of financial resources.

So, if each patient is provided with one hour of education group per day at thirty dollars for three days each week, that represents ninety dollars per week per patient. Add to that, each patient will receive six hours of group therapy at thirty dollars per hour, which comes to $180. Each patient will also receive one hour of individual therapy at sixty-five dollars. So the total income generated by providing ten hours of treatment services for one week is $90 + $180 + $65 = $335.

The average cost to the patient for two and a half hours of treatment services per day is $83.75. This is a bargain.

Okay, you say that a program cannot support itself by charging so little for it services. Well, let us see.

You have four licensed counselors who can easily manage a caseload of at least eight patients. With that in mind, each counselor's caseload generates a program income of $2,680 per week. Therefore, four counselors' caseloads combined represent an income of $10,720 per week.

Let us also assume that the program operates for forty-eight weeks out of fifty-two weeks that are available during the year. That allows personnel two weeks annual vacation, one week for professional training, and one week during the Christmas holiday. Nobody wants to be in treatment at Christmas!

Then, an income of $10,720 per week for forty-eight weeks generates an annual income of $514,560. With an operating budget of $350,000 and an actual income of $514,560, there is a profit of $164,560 for this small program. This is profit that can be utilized to cover unexpected expense and the purchase of additional materials. This profit could also be applied to expansion of services and facilities, or it can be held in reserve.

This is a simplified example. Nevertheless, it does illustrate that a small intensive outpatient program can support itself while at the same time providing cost-effective treatment services. Granted, no one is going to get rich working in such a program. But, who gets rich when traditional inpatient programs charge about ten thousand dollars, or more, per week? It's not the program's staff!

Program Staff. Thus far, we have discussed treatment settings (inpatient versus intensive outpatient), facility requirements, and cost efficiency. Another extremely important consideration is who will be providing the treatment services. Relying on our hypothetical small program wherein there is one program director, four counselors, two education specialists, and one clerical/support person, let us examine the qualifications we need to provide quality addictions treatment.

In Chapter Six, there was an extensive discussion regarding the lack of professional qualifications among typical addictions counselors. Often, counselors in traditional addictions treatment programs may not have a four-year college degree in any behavioral science. Many of these same counselors are individuals who are in recovery from their own addictions and decide to aid others with substance use problems. Eligibility for certification or licensure as an addictions counselor in many jurisdictions requires that an individual receive an education approximately equivalent to six or seven undergraduate college classes, along with approximately two years supervised experience in the provision of addictions treatment services.

Experience, both in the form of recovery from one's own problems and from helping others do the same, is valuable in the development of a counselor's professional qualifications. However, if that experience is not coupled with an education that provides for a thorough understanding of human behavior and of mental illness, it's not likely that a prospective counselor will be sufficiently prepared to effectively deal with mental illness as it is manifested in the form of a substance use disorder.

Previously, the question was posed: for what other mental disorder would we presume that a person who has taken the equivalent of six or seven college classes, and has three years of exposure to one approach to treating any disorder, would be qualified to provide effective treatment? The answer is: only in the addictions treatment industry! Much of the education and experience that these addictions counselors do receive is centered on the "disease concept" and twelve-step methodology. It's no mystery why traditional treatment for substance use disorders has never established a demonstrable record for success.

Any individual who provides direct treatment services to people suffering from mental illness, including substance use disorders, should be appropriately qualified. In almost any jurisdiction in this nation, that means that a counselor, therapist, or licensed practioner would need to have a master's degree in a behavioral science, such as clinical psychology or counseling psychology, from a fully accredited college or university. In addition to the education requirement, most jurisdictions also require a minimum of one year of supervised experience in the provision of treatment services to become eligible for licensure or certification.

The substance abuse disorders are recognized mental illnesses. This is why they are listed among all other recognized mental illnesses in the *Diagnostic and Statistical Manual of Mental Disorders, Fourth Edition* (APA, 1994). While substance use disorders are not more difficult to understand or to treat, they certainly are not less complex than other mental disorders. Why on earth could we have ever imagined that individuals who have little education related to the understanding of mental illness would be capable of effectively treating individuals who suffer from any recognized mental illness? Seventy years of failure in the provision of addictions treatment should demonstrate that they cannot.

I take a firm stance on the proposition that those who provide direct treatment services, such as individual and group therapy, should be appropriately qualified to do so. Therefore, individuals designated as counselors in any substance abuse treatment setting should be masters-level counselors.

In our hypothetical program, there are four counselors. These individuals would manage and provide each patient's treatment. In this program, the counselors would specifically be assigned to provide their patients with individual and group therapy.

As outlined, there were also two education specialists. These two individuals would be assigned the task of providing patients with the psycho-educational services. In this hypothetical treatment program, these services would be provided in a group setting similar to a classroom setting. Essentially this is an effort to educate patients regarding their illness and its associated problems and to assist patients in the acquisition of the skills needed to have a real chance to overcome their disorder. The exact content of this education will be discussed more thoroughly later.

Educational specialists are basically teachers. As such, individuals who are assigned these educational tasks should be appropriately qualified as well. It may not be necessary for these individuals to be certified teachers, but the educational qualifications should be similar. I propose that educational specialists should be required to have a bachelor's degree from an accredited college or university with a major field of study in a recognized behavioral science. Such an educational foundation would provide these specialists with the skills needed to impart beneficial information to patients.

The director in our proposed program would have to perform two primary roles. The first role would be that of a clinical director. That is, the program director would assume overall responsibility for the treatment provided. The director would also be responsible for the administration of fiscal and human resources. The specific qualifications of the program director would need to appear to be quite divergent and disparate. To some extent, this is true. However, this is a *treatment* program. All activity is to be devoted to the provision of services benefiting others. It is not a corporate business venture intended only to generate income. The primary role of the director is to ensure that the treatment offered is effective. As such, the director must be a qualified clinician. The director must have the ability to structure treatment services to make these services effective. This can only be accomplished if the director has a thorough understanding of mental illness and the treatment of mental illnesses. Therefore, the program director must be a masters-level licensed therapist, at minimum. Without such qualifications, the director will not have the ability to offer instruction and guidance to counselors and educational specialists.

Additionally, the director will also have to the ability to take on such tasks as budgeting, allocating program resources, billing for services, collection of income, quality control, program planning, managing personnel, etc. These additional duties sound overwhelming, don't they? If an individual has attained the personal discipline required to become a licensed therapist, learning the skills required to take on these additional duties is certainly possible. Remember, this is a small program of simple design. If implemented appropriately, much of the activity required to carry out these administrative activities can simply be designed into the core of the activities carried on within the program on a daily basis. Certainly, the program director should be an individual with some administrative experience and some additional education related to business and agency administration. I believe that the most important qualification that an individual assuming the position of program director should possess is the ability and willingness to lead.

Last but not least is the clerical support position. While this position is not clinical in nature, it is nonetheless an important role that must be carried out in a professional and disciplined manner if the overall program is to run efficiently. Clerical support is a position that wears many hats. This individual may act as the program's receptionist and as a clerical assistant to the program director. The clerical support person must be skilled in verbal and written communication. This individual must also be able to get along well with others. The person who fulfills the clerical support position within the program should have attained, at least, a high school education, and should also have some additional education in business or secretarial skills.

There it is. A treatment program is really only as good as those who carry out the activities related to the provision of treatment services. As such, much care should be given to the selection of individuals whose education and experience provides them with a knowledge base that promotes the potential for success.

Historically, the addictions treatment industry has not required that those who provide treatment services have any formal and specific education and experience in understanding and treating mental illness. The primary qualification of an addictions counselor is that he or she should be in recovery, according to twelve-step thinking, along with having some education related to the behavioral sciences.

Duration of Treatment. How long does it take to definitively treat a substance use disorder, and just how many hours of group and individual therapy does that entail? The popular answer to this compound question is that it takes approximately thirty-four hours of a combination of group and individual counseling over a period of exactly twenty-eight days to definitively treat a substance use disorder. This has been the correct answer for the last forty years, according to our existing addictions treatment industry. Well, that was easy, wasn't it?

Oh, darn! I forgot a few things. We had better qualify that answer in a couple of ways. According to the evidence to date, this correctly answers the question for about five percent of those individuals who partake of existing treatment (Bufe, 1998). Only about 16 percent of the people who suffer from a substance use disorder ever seek formal treatment for their problems (SAMSHA, 2000). It appears as though the correct answer is not true for the overwhelming majority of individuals who suffer from substance use disorders.

How has it been determined that the provision of twenty-eight days of minimal intervention should be sufficient as an effort to definitively treat substance use disorders?

If you will recall from our earlier discussions related to the evolution of the addictions treatment industry (see Chapter Four), traditional twelve-step treatment was given a tremendous impetus for development as a result of the passage of the Hughes Act in 1970. This indirectly paved the way for encouraging private insurance companies to provide coverage for twelve-step inpatient treatment. As larger sums of money became available to pay for addictions treatment subsequent to the passage of that act, corporate enterprises, primarily in the form of large, corporate hospitals and other health-care enterprises, began to recognize that there might be great profit potential in offering inpatient treatment for alcoholism and drug addictions. Thus, there was a literal nationwide explosion in the creation of addictions treatment programs during the 1970s and 1980s. It seemed that everybody wanted to get in on the twelve-step treatment boom.

However, by the late 1980s, private insurers and managed-care organizations became increasingly reluctant to pay for traditional inpatient treatment simply because there had never been any demonstration that inpatient treatment resulted in any better outcomes than other outpatient treatment efforts. Ultimately, private insurers began to place limitations on what they were willing to pay out for inpatient treatment (Nace, 1993; Schmidt and Wiesner, 1993). Payment limitations, in turn, resulted in shorter stays for patients seeking inpatient treatment.

The standard of twenty-eight days of inpatient treatment has nothing to do with whether this is the actual amount of treatment required to definitively treat addictions. It's all about payment and profits. Simply, inpatient treatment programs have recognized that health insurance companies will only pay for up to twenty-eight days of inpatient treatment. Magically, at the end of twenty-eight days, patients are cured; they are ready to face the real world without continued reliance upon mood-altering substances. This is not, overall, a realistic expectation. As has been demonstrated, this is realistic about 5 percent of the time.

Once again the question is posed: how long does it take to definitively treat someone who suffers from a substance use disorder, and just how many hours of group and individual therapy does that entail? I propose the following as the best available answer to this question: *It takes as much time as it takes, and it entails as much individual and group therapy as it takes to reasonably ensure that the substance-abusing patient has developed the skills needed to adapt to daily living without relying upon the use of mood-altering substances to cope with the challenges of daily living.*

Treatment for addictions, regardless of the approach or the treatment setting, needs to be open-ended. The notion that a set amount of treatment will result in the individual overcoming a substance use problem or other mental disorder is patently absurd. Time limits for the treatment of mental disorders are nothing more than arbitrary limitations set by accountants.

The onset for substance use problems is insidious. For most individuals, these problems have developed over many years, sometimes over an entire lifetime. It is not reasonable to assume that these problems can be alleviated in a matter of days, a few weeks, or even over a few months in some cases. The truth is that many individuals who suffer from substance use disorders struggle for many years until they find exactly the type of assistance needed to help them overcome their substance abuse problems.

The word of caution that I would extend to anyone who might attempt to design and implement services that are to be devoted to the treatment of substance use disorders is to create an approach that is open-ended. There is nothing wrong with estimating the amount of time or services needed to be successful in treating an average patient. However, with respect to any estimate, it is wise to remain mindful that the actual amount of time that will be need to be devoted to a successful treatment effort will vary a great deal from one patient to another.

It takes what it takes! No more. No less.

We have now discussed some of the more important foundational considerations in any attempt to create an effective and cost-efficient treatment effort. This is, by no means, intended to represent a detailed listing of all that must be given attention when assuming the task of designing and implementing an addictions treatment effort. Yet, paying close attention to considerations, such as specific treatment settings, facility requirements, qualifications of treatment personnel, costs, and treatment duration, will go a long way in ensuring that the treatment services will rest on a solid foundation.

References

Chapter Twelve

Alcoholics Anonymous World Services (1980). *Dr. Bob and the Good Oldtimers.* (p. 83) New York, NY.

American Psychiatric Association (1994). *Diagnostic and Statistical Manual of Mental Disorders, Fourth Edition.* Washington, DC.

Bufe, C. (1998). How effective is AA? *Alcoholics Anonymous: Cult or Cure.* 2nd Edition, revised. San Francisco, CA: See Sharp Press.

Holden, C. (1987). Is alcoholism treatment effective? *Science,* **236,** 20–22.

Miller, W. R., and Hester, R. K. (1986). Inpatient alcoholism treatment: Who benefits? *American Psychologist,* **41,** 794–805.

Mojtabai, R., and Zivin, J. G. (2003). Effectiveness and cost-effectiveness of four treatment modalities for substance disorders: A propensity score analysis. *Health Education Research,* **38(1),** 233–2597.

Nace, E. (1993). Inpatient treatment. Marc Galanter, (Ed.), *Recent Developments in Alcoholism, Volume 11: Ten Years of Progress.* New York, NY: Plenum Press.

Nathan, P. E., and Skinstad, A. (1987). Outcomes of treatment for alcohol problems: Current methods, problems, and results. *Journal of Consulting and Clinical Psychology,* **55,** 332–340.

Schmidt, L., and Weisner, C. (1993). Developments in alcoholism treatment. M. Galanter, (Ed.), *Recent Developments in*

Alcoholism, Volume 11: Ten Years of Progress (p. 374). New York, NY: Plenum Press.

Substance Abuse and Mental Health Services Administration (2000). National Household Survey on Drug Abuse, 2000. Office of Applied Studies. Web site: http://www.oas.samhsa.gov.

Roman, P., and Blum, T. (1997). National treatment center study six and twelve month follow-up summary report. (Table 11, p. 47). Athens, GA: Institute for Behavioral Research.

Weithmann, G., and Hoffmann, M. (2005). A randomized clinical trial of in-patient versus combined day hospital treatment of alcoholism: Primary and secondary outcome measures. *European Addiction Research,* **11(4)**, 197–203.

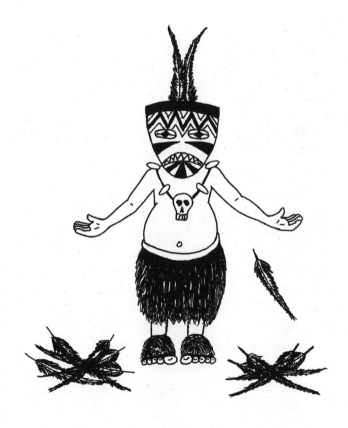

Chapter 13

Treatment Goals

I believe that the treatment of substance use disorders is best undertaken via a team approach. It truly takes a comprehensive and intensive treatment effort to achieve a specific set of short-term goals and objectives that are the keys to assisting the substance-abusing patients to attain the overall goal of treatment: abandoning the abuse of mood-altering substances while learning more appropriate and constructive behaviors. This must be accomplished in as short a period of time as possible.

When treating any mental disorder, the more quickly an individual can experience positive outcomes as a result of his or her involvement, the more likely it is that the individual will adhere to the treatment effort. In other words, patients want results. Therefore, a comprehensive and intensive treatment effort which attempts to attain target-specific treatment goals and objectives in short order is most likely to engender patient confidence and cooperation.

Treatment for substance use disorders can have only one ultimate goal: for the substance abusing patient to abandon the use of alcohol and/or drugs in favor of learning and implementing more effective and constructive means of coping. In order to achieve such an ultimate goal in a relatively short period of time, I believe that there exists a specific set of general objectives or short term goals (STG) that all substance-abusing patients must strive to achieve while they are involved in treatment. These short term goals are: 1) the patient must continue to constructively address the denial of personal problems; 2) the patient must acknowledge the connection existing between the use of mood-altering substances and the desire to escape troublesome thoughts and emotions; 3) the patient must learn and implement new, more effective, and constructive strategies for dealing with troublesome thoughts and emotions; and 4) the patient must create a balanced lifestyle.

This may appear to be a rather simplistic set of goals for treatment. However, as will be demonstrated, the attainment of these short term goals will require a substantial amount of work on the parts of both the patients and the treatment providers. Let us now take a look at what must be accomplished to facilitate the patient's attainment of each of these goals.

STG #1: Constructively addressing ongoing denial

The traditional approach to addictions treatment has held denial to be the "cardinal and integral feature of chemical dependency and the fatal aspect of alcoholism and other drug dependencies" (Hazelden, 1975, p. 9). In keeping with this perspective, traditional treatment approaches have also conveniently used patient denial as the primary explanation as to why patients fail in treatment. That is, if the patient lacks motivation, fails to comply with treatment recommendations, leaves treatment prior to completion, or fails to enter treatment at all, it is because the patient is in denial.

Now, this is circular logic. Let's examine this proposition. The patient has a disease of which denial is a "cardinal and integral feature." In order for the patient to overcome or control this disease, the patient must undergo traditional treatment wherein the patient's denial will be aggressively and exhaustingly confronted. Then, if the patient fails to overcome or control the disease after having been exposed to such treatment, which we already know is more often the case than not, it's because the patient has a disease causing the patient to be in denial. Precisely, the reason that the treatment for the disease fails is because the patient has the disease. How much sense does this make?

Chapter Eleven is devoted to how traditional twelve-step treatment has insanely misused the concept of denial. I hope to offer the reader a more reasonable and therapeutic approach to addressing patient denial.

Denial is a psychological defense against fear and uncertainty. Patients exhibit denial in many ways. In most instances, patients exhibit this fear and uncertainty by being hesitant to actively engage in prescribed activities. Most therapists call this hesitance on the part of their patients' resistance. Patients resist what is asked of them because they are fearful and uncertain of the outcome. Individuals who have become accustomed to using alcohol and/or drugs as a primary means of coping are fearful of abandoning such practices, as they know no other effective means of coping. Additionally, they would be uncertain of how they will cope without the use of mood-altering substances.

Aggressive confrontation of the substance-abusing patient's denial or resistance which has been characteristic of traditional twelve-step treatment approaches has never been demonstrated to be therapeutic (Lieberman et al., 1973; MacDonough, 1976; Miller et al., 1993). Such confrontation will only add to the patient's fear and uncertainty, thereby causing the patient to become more resistant and much more defensive. The most natural response that any patient will have to being aggressively and exhaustingly confronted about fearsome issues and circumstances is to deny their existence. Aggressive confrontation of patient denial only perpetuates the patient's problems, driving the patient even deeper into a state of denial wherein he or she will be forced to adopt an assortment of defensive positions.

Still, this denial and resistance are real issues which must be resolved so that the patient can actively engage in therapy and make progress toward the attainment of therapeutic goals and objectives. How does a therapist approach denial without driving the patient even deeper into this defensive posture?

When attempting to assist a patient with denial, it is always important for the therapist, or any treatment provider, to approach the patient in a nonjudgmental and nonthreatening manner. In the early stages of treatment, the patient is just beginning to develop a trusting relationship with the therapist. Trust is a condition that must be earned, not forced. Therefore, counselors and therapists must be willing to create an environment which conveys an acceptance of the patient. Being accepting of the patient does not equate to offering approval for the patient's exhibition of inappropriate and destructive behavior. It simply means that the treatment providers must approach the patient in ways that acknowledge the patient's right to be treated with dignity and respect. Carl Rogers (1959) described this as affording the patient "unconditional positive regard."

Treatment professionals must anticipate that denial is ever present in addictions treatment, just as it is in the treatment of any other disorder. As soon as any patient is confronted with a thought, emotion, issue, or set of circumstances which he or she has been unable to constructively address, it is possible that the patient will deny that such a problem might exist. Consequently, the patient may try to avoid any attempt on the part of the therapist to introduce the problem as a topic that is open to discussion.

Therapists who are adequately trained and experienced in the provision of treatment services quickly recognize patient denial and other forms of psychological defense. Therapists who have significant experience in working with substance-using patients understand that a patient's denial indicates a problem that is contributing to the use of mood-altering substances. The patient's denial has just served as a signal to the therapist that the problem introduced for discussion is likely a problem which has historically caused this patient to experience fear and uncertainty. The patient has never been able to find an effective and constructive means of dealing with this problem. In turn, this thought, emotion, issue, or set of circumstances is likely to trigger the patient's desire to use mood-altering substances as a means of alleviating the fear and uncertainty the patient experiences with every confrontation.

In a roundabout way, patient denial is a therapeutic doorway into what can be, metaphorically, described as a disorderly storage closet likely to contain all sorts of problems. Some of those problems may be directly related to the patient's substance use, some may not. Once the therapist has knocked on that door, and the patient has denied initial entry, the therapist must eventually gain access to this closet to help the patient find a more effective and constructive way to clean up the disorder. With regard to treatment of addictions, how does the therapist quickly gain access through this doorway of denial to help the patient?

The aggressive and relentless confrontation characteristic of traditional twelve-step treatment efforts is seldom beneficial to the patient in any way. The harder the therapist pounds on the door, the more resistance the patient will exhibit to block admission.

Earlier a reference was made to Carl Rogers's concept of "unconditional positive regard." I fully believe that the only way a therapist can gain admission into the areas of the patient's life wherein denial remains an obstacle is to genuinely convey "unconditional positive regard" to the patient.

Let's take a few moments to examine exactly what is meant by unconditional positive regard (UPR). Rogers (1959) offers an extremely good definition of this concept.

> *Unconditional*—One experiencing UPR holds "no conditions of acceptance.... It is at the opposite pole from a selective evaluating attitude." (p.225)

> *Positive*—One offers "warm acceptance ... a prizing of the person, as Dewey has used the term.... It means caring for the client." (p. 225)

> *Regard*—One regards "each aspect of the client, but not in a possessive way or in such a way as simply to satisfy the therapists own needs. It means caring for the client as a separate person, with permission to have his [or her] own feelings, his [or her] own experiences." (p. 225)

In other words, UPR means that a therapist must attempt to approach his or her work with any given patient in a manner which conveys a willingness to be caring and accepting of the patient. This must be done even if that given patient does not for the moment feel or think about the issues at hand in the same way as the therapist does.

This is not what happens in traditional twelve-step treatment for addictions. In that setting, acceptance of the patient is predicated upon whether or not the patient is willing to readily admit that he or she is in denial as it is defined within twelve-step ideology. If a patient can be psychologically coerced into verbally admitting to his or her problem(s), most often within the context of a group therapy setting, whether or not the patient actually perceives the problems in the same way as does the therapist, only then is the patient offered positive regard.

Matters are made even worse by the fact that such selective evaluations of the patient on the part of traditional treatment providers are purely subjective in nature. There is no reliable way to accurately and objectively measure denial. Worse yet is that these subjective evaluations are made by individuals who often lack any qualifications to make accurate judgments.

There is much truth in the adage that you can attract more flies with honey than with vinegar. It has been my experience that a patient, in any treatment setting, is much more willing to trust therapists and other treatment providers if it is the patient's perception that the service providers genuinely care for the patient's well-being, accepts the patient as a human being despite his or her imperfections, and grants the patient the dignity and respect that should be afforded to any other person. When a patient trusts the motives of the therapist and believes that the therapist is not passing judgment on every word and action, there is no reason for the patient to resist the therapist's effort to explore potential problem areas. After all, denial is simply a defense against perceived threat.

The key that unlocks this metaphorical doorway to the closet that holds whatever a given patient regards with fear and uncertainty is trust. A therapist or other treatment provider who offers the patient unconditional positive regard will inevitably engender the patient's trust. This, in turn, will result in much less resistance and denial on the part of the patient. It will allow for an environment wherein the patient will not so actively resist the therapist's attempt to gain a glimpse of what exists behind the door.

Let's take another look at our short-term treatment goal relating to denial. STG #1: *The patient must continue to constructively address denial of personal problems.*

This goal, as it is stated, does not mean that our treatment should be directed toward eliminating patient denial. Even if this could be accomplished in some way, this is simply not an option for any ethical and competent treatment provider. Our goal is merely to assist our substance-using patient in recognizing and acknowledging existing problems, and seeing these problems in less psychologically threatening ways. The objective is to help the patient see problems as issues that can be faced or, at the very least, minimized in terms of the negative impact that the given problem might have of on the patient's life.

The aggressive and exhausting confrontation typical in traditional twelve-step treatment, using the patient's problems as an emotional bludgeon to coerce the patient into seeing his or her problems the way that the counselor sees them, is not even remotely related to the achievement of this goal. A therapist or other treatment provider who would utilize such approaches is really more interested in using the patient to affirm the treatment provider's personal world view than in helping the patient.

As was stated in prior sections, denial and other psychological defenses are ever present in any treatment setting. It is never appropriate, nor is it in any way constructive, for a therapist or any other treatment provider to eliminate a patient's psychological defenses. It is the treatment professional's obligation to assist the patient in learning to see problems from new and various perspectives and to teach the patient alternative ways to resolve some of the problems that the patient must face. Offering the patient "unconditional positive regard" is the only avenue that leads to the attainment of the goal of having the patient continue to constructively address denial.

Once a patient behaviorally exhibits the willingness to acknowledge the existence of the offending problem, denial has been adequately and constructively addressed! This behavioral exhibition of willingness on the part of the patient can take the form of allowing the therapist to calmly and dispassionately engage in a discussion of the suspected problem. It does not require that a patient must immediately adopt the same perspective regarding the problem as that held by the therapist. It is the therapist's responsibility to see the problem as the patient does, not the other way around.

Successful treatment providers do not attempt to judge, condemn, or indoctrinate; they merely align with their patients to introduce new potentials and possibilities. The tools needed to achieve such an alignment are genuine empathy and a willingness to suspend any judgments they might make based on personally held beliefs and biases.

STG #2: The patient must acknowledge the connection existing between the use of mood-altering substances and the desire to escape troublesome thoughts and emotions.

Alcohol and other drugs do not spontaneously possess the mind and soul of any individual, nor is addiction the result of being singled out by God to be genetically or biochemically defective and, therefore, intensely vulnerable to the evil nature of mood-altering substances. Such anthropomorphication of alcohol and drugs, combined with the fatalistic thinking which is ever-present in modern twelve-step ideology, has never been a tenable position from which treatment for addictions can be initiated.

An individual becomes psychologically, and sometimes physically, reliant upon alcohol and other mood-altering chemicals for a reason. The reason for this reliance is that these substances offer the individual a readily accessible means of escaping personal discomfort.

Personal discomfort comes in many forms. Discomfort can be psychological in that it results from an individual's way of thinking and/or feeling. Discomfort can be the result of the individual's experience of actual physical pain, or it can result from a combination of these two sources. In some instances, even the mere anticipation of real or imagined discomfort can provide an individual with the motivation to escape this perceived threat by using mood-altering substances.

The *only* reason that any individual engages in the habitual use of mood-altering substances is exactly as the term "mood-altering" implies. The individual engages in this escapist, avoidant behavior to change his or her mood. Mood is defined in *Webster's II New Riverside Dictionary* (1984) as: "1. a temporary state of emotion or mind: feeling; 2. prevailing spirit: disposition."

A person's mood directly represents how the self is perceived in relation to the surrounding world. If a person is experiencing a good mood, or even just a stable mood, this is a presentation indicating that the individual's perceptions of this relationship are acceptable. The person perceives that his or her existence is safe and tolerable. On the other hand, a negative or unstable mood indicates that the individual's perceived well-being is in some way in jeopardy. Increasingly, individuals living in our modern society find this latter state of thinking and feeling to be intolerable. Because of a negative or unstable mood, the individual is most likely to attempt to modify the negative mood through the use of a mood-altering chemical.

Mood-altering chemicals, such as alcohol, marijuana, cocaine, heroin, and so on, are very effective when used as a means to change an individual's immediate state of thinking and feeling. A few beers, a few hits, a line or two, or whatever is all that is needed to temporarily change an individual's state of thinking and feeling from being bad to good, great, or even glorious. If this use of mood-altering chemicals to alter one's state of mind is repeated, eventually use will become habitual.

In a previous chapter, I offered the following definition of substance dependence:

> *Substance dependence represents a psychological, and sometimes physiological, reliance upon a given mood-altering substance that serves an adaptive and defensive function in response to a real or perceived need or an existing coping deficit for which the individual has not yet developed the specific skills or learned the appropriate functional behaviors needed to fulfill this need or to correct the deficit in a more effective and constructive manner. This reliance will result in the repetitious use of mood-altering substances that will endure until such a time when the individual develops the skills or learns the appropriate behaviors needed to fulfill his or her need or correct an existing deficit in a more effective and constructive manner.*

At this point, I would like to take a few moments to further explain why I believe this definition is much more meaningful to the treatment of addictions than past definitions. This definition explains the habitual use of mood-altering substances in terms of *purpose-driven behavior*. Individuals engage in the complex behaviors of ingesting, smoking, inhaling, or injecting a mood-altering substance, or a variety of substances, for the purpose of responding to a perceived need to effect a positive change in the way the individual is experiencing his or her immediate existence.

Behavior is observable. We can see it. We can, at the very least, approximate a reasonable understanding of it. We can even quantify it if we must. More importantly, for the purpose of treatment, we can alter behavior.

Defining substance dependence as the result of an individual's genetic makeup or as abnormal neuro-biochemical processes gives us little to correct. First, if we believe that substance dependence is the result of genetic abnormality, we must admit that there is no consensus as to what part of an individual's genetic makeup should be regarded as being abnormal, or how that abnormality causes the habitual use of mood-altering substances. Which chromosome or chromosomal pairing is connected to substance-abusing behavior, and how does this make an individual use mood-altering substances? Even if the answers to these important questions could be proven, what could we do to effect a change?

Second, if we assume that substance-abusing behavior is caused by a neuro-biochemical abnormality, which chemicals or neurotransmitters are actually involved? Research, to date, has hypothetically connected the use of mood-altering substances to nearly every chemical within our brains! Do abnormalities in the dopaminergic neurotransmission systems cause an individual to use mood-altering chemicals? How about those systems which operate primarily in response to serotonin? How about the endorphins? Which chemical? What crucial difference in chemical levels or pathways exists? More importantly, what can we do to effect a change in any or all of this today?

There is one thing that all of us can agree upon today: the use of mood-altering substances is a behavior. And, as Pavlov (1927) and Watson (1929) clearly demonstrated many years ago, *behavior can be changed*. Changing this behavior is probable when we understand

271

that individuals engage in the use of mood-altering substances for readily evident reasons.

By the time work on STG #2 begins, the patient's treatment team should already have a relatively good idea as to why the patient has been using mood-altering substances. The patient has undergone medical, psychological, and social assessments, an alcohol and drug use history has been complied, and it is likely that the treatment team has gathered other collateral information relevant to the patient's life history as well. This has been done to devise an operational conceptualization of the patient's substance use problem(s) as was outlined in Chapter Seven.

By now, the team members should have a reasonably accurate understanding of why the patient is reliant upon the use of mood-altering chemicals to escape or avoid specific problems. Because they have operationally defined the patient's problem(s), the team can design a treatment approach specifically targeting the patient's reasons for using these substances.

As important as this understanding is to those who provide treatment services, it is equally important to the patient. The patient must recognize that reliance upon alcohol or drugs is directly connected to an inability to effectively and constructively cope with problematic thoughts and emotions.

How does the treatment team help patients make this connection?

One simple way is to ask the patient why he or she uses alcohol or drugs. Amazing! As treatment experts, we might actually learn about the patient's perceptions regarding substance use simply by asking. Even more amazing is that the individual will almost always tell us precisely why he or she engages in the use of alcohol and/or drugs.

For twenty years, I have always made it a point to ask each and every patient to tell me why he or she uses alcohol and/or drugs. Few individuals could not provide a reasonable explanation as to why they needed to use these substances. What is truly astonishing is that the reasons articulated by these patients have been remarkably similar! Certainly the responses offered from one individual to another have varied. Some have stated that they use to ward off feelings of depression or sad memories. Some have stated that they use to feel more social. Some say they use to relax. Some have indicated that fear is what causes them to seek comfort in the use of alcohol or drugs. Some have cited anger as the reason. Some have stated that they use to escape boredom. Some have even stated that they use because they like the sensation.

Do you see a common thread here? Depression, anxiety, anger, social unease, boredom, and even a desire to feel better are all commonly regarded as negative emotions. All are emotional states to avoid whenever possible. So, what is common to all individuals who use abuse alcohol and/or drugs? They all do so to avoid or escape uncomfortable thoughts and feelings.

In addition to simply asking why a patient uses alcohol and/or drugs, there are numerous other methods to aid treatment providers in their efforts to assist the patient in gaining insight as to why the patient has come to rely upon mood-altering chemicals as a means of escaping or avoiding specific thoughts and feelings. The specific method chosen should depend upon the needs of the patient. Consideration should always be given to understanding how each patient relates to the world. We will talk more about this later.

For now, we are talking about simply achieving our second short-term goal. To sum it all up, the habitual use of mood-altering chemicals represents a specific type of behavior. This behavior serves a functional and adaptive purpose for the individual. Behavior can be changed.

Now, how does all this apply to our second short-term treatment goal? Again, STG #2 says the patient must acknowledge the connection between the use of mood-altering substances and the desire to escape troublesome thoughts and emotions. When treatment providers can move the patient toward the achievement of this STG, two important aspects of the patient's substance use problems become clear to both patient and provider. When this STG is achieved, the patient and the provider have gained significant insight into *what* the problem is— *what* as it relates to substance dependence is the behavior including habitual use of mood-altering chemicals. The second aspect is *why* the patient engages in this behavior. The patient and treatment team have gained significant insight as to the functional and adaptive purpose for the patient's use of mood-altering substances.

Now that the patient and the treatment team have come to a clear understanding as to what behavior needs to be changed and why it occurred, the next logical short-term goal should consist of helping the patient to devise more effective and constructive behaviors as a means of coping with discomfort.

STG #3: The patient must learn and implement new, more effective, and constructive strategies for dealing with troublesome thoughts and emotions.

By the time a patient becomes ready to attempt this third STG, several significant events have occurred as a result of the patient's participation in the treatment effort. First, the patient has acknowledged that he or she has become reliant upon mood-altering substances and that this reliance represents a real threat to the patient's physical and mental health. The patient has also acknowledged that a continued reliance may cause a whole host of significant personal and social problems. Second, the patient has gained insight as to the reason for this reliance. The patient has gained awareness that using these mood-altering substances was an attempt to escape or avoid negative thoughts and emotions.

To follow the logic forming the foundation of the treatment approach I am advocating, I will once again restate my definition of substance dependence:

> *Substance dependence represents a psychological, and sometimes physiological, reliance upon a given mood-altering substance that serves an adaptive and defensive function in response to a real or perceived need or an existing coping deficit for which the individual has not yet developed the specific skills or learned the appropriate functional behaviors needed to fulfill this need or to correct the deficit in a more effective and constructive manner. This reliance will result in the repetitious use of mood-altering substances that will endure until such time as the individual develops the skills or learns the appropriate behaviors needed to fulfill his or her*

need or correct an existing deficit in a more effective and constructive manner.

When the treatment team has assisted a substance-abusing patient to achieve, or even approximate, the first two short-term goals, the patient has made significant headway in overcoming his or her problem. The patient has addressed denial to a point where there is an acknowledgement of a reliance on mood-altering substances which is a problem.

However, what distinguishes this treatment approach from approaches having faith in the disease concept of addiction is that this approach alerts the patient to the concept that there is an actual reason for the reliance. More importantly, it's a reason that the patient can address directly.

The patient is not asked to accept that he or she has no control over a mythical disease with an unfounded genetic or biochemical cause. The patient has learned that the use of mood-altering chemicals is a response to a real human need. That's right; the patient has learned that his or her behavior, as dysfunctional and destructive as it might have been, has actually served an adaptive and functional purpose.

The patient is not led to believe that he or she has been singled out by God and rendered genetically or biochemically abnormal. This, by the way, would be an abnormality undefined. The patient is not asked to announce that he or she is insane. The patient is not told to turn his or her will over to some ambiguously defined God in the hope that He will somehow return the patient to a state of wholeness. The patient is not told that the only hope of salvation relies on a willingness to adhere to a specific set of steps nor that the patient must attend meetings for the rest of his or her natural life.

Instead of being asked to rely on God, as His goodwill toward alcoholics and drug addicts is only manifested to souls affiliated with AA or NCADD, what would a patient participating in the treatment approach using short-term goals one and two do to get better?

The patient would learn new skills!

What? That's it? All they need to do is learn some skills in order to get better?

Yes, the answer is that simple! All that a substance-abusing patient needs to do to change destructive behavior is to learn skills that more directly and constructively fulfill needs. The patient needs to learn what to do *instead* of turning to the use of mood-altering chemicals! It is that simple. Of course, simplicity does not necessarily equate with ease.

Substance abusers do not share a common personality type. There is no such thing as an addictive personality. Stating that personality is the culprit in the development of substance use disorders is no different from assigning the blame to genetics or neurochemistry. We really don't know that any such assertions are true, and we certainly cannot demonstrate that adherence to these ideas is helpful to the patient.

Additionally, while many substance abusing persons do appear to suffer similar kinds of psychological problems, such as depression, anxiety, impulsivity, and anger, etc., the mere fact that individuals may suffer from one or more of these problems has not proven to be predictive of any predisposition to engage in the use of mood-altering chemicals. We do know that there exists many more individuals, from all nations and walks of life, who encounter such problems in the course of their lives without becoming reliant upon mood-altering chemicals than there are individuals who do turn to the use of drugs and/or alcohol. So, if abnormalities related to genetics, neurochemistry, personality, or the existence of psychological problems cannot singularly account for an individual's tendency to become reliant upon mood-altering chemicals to escape personal discomfort, what can possibly account for the use of drugs and/or alcohol?

What I have observed is that almost all substance-dependent individuals exhibit noticeably immature behavior, which is indicative of an underdeveloped sense of self. Their behavior, in almost all cases, indicates that such individuals are deficient in appropriate socialization; they exhibit poor impulse control; and they exhibit an obvious inability to accurately interpret objective reality. Substance-abusing patients also tend to exhibit extreme self-centeredness and poor insight into their own behavior; plus they are unable to tolerate unpleasant thoughts and feelings.

As can be seen, what is being stressed is not that substance-dependent individuals all share a common pathology related to genetics, neurochemistry, or even personality. What is being stressed is that the behavior exhibited by these individuals is noticeably immature or underdeveloped.

I believe that substance-abusing behavior is more a developmental issue than it is an issue related to genetics, neurochemistry, or personality. Substance-abusing individuals do not suffer from any abnormality in their genetic makeup, neurochemistry, or personality causing a predisposition to the use of mood-altering chemicals. Research to date has never demonstrated that such abnormality exists. Essentially, something can't be considered to be broken, or abnormal, if it was never there to begin with!

What is observable in the behavior of any substance-abusing person is that this person never learned how to deal with life's complexities and challenges in a normal, mature manner. Instead of developing the skills to effectively and constructively deal with life's challenges, substance-abusing persons have learned to use alcohol and/or drugs. Simply stated, substance-abusing individuals are developmentally immature.

This may seem like a very bold and sweeping statement. In some respects, I will admit that it is. But, let's examine more closely what is being stated here.

To be considered to be mature, according to *Webster's New Riverside Dictionary* (1984, p. 431), an individual must have, "1. attained full growth and development; 2. exhibit the characteristics associated with an adult." Conversely, to be considered immature or underdeveloped, Webster's (p. 746) states that the individual has "not developed in a full or normal way."

When we as clinicians closely examine the medical, psychological, and social histories compiled to formulate an operational conceptualization of our patients' problems, it should be obvious that each one of our substance-abusing patients share something. What all these patients have in common is not that they each have similar genetic traits, aside from their being genetically identifiable as human beings, nor is it that each one of these individuals has a brain that functions, neuro-chemically, in an identical manner. What all our patients do have in common is that they each have experienced identifiable events and/or circumstances preventing them from developing fully or normally.

Unlike other creatures that inhabit this planet, human beings are born with very few innate instincts or tendencies to survive. We are not born with the ability to swim, to walk and talk, to seek out and secure sources of food and shelter. We are not even born with the ability to distinguish danger from safety. Human beings must learn all of these skills to survive.

Some have even suggested that when human beings enter this life, each exists as a veritable blank slate. In 1690, the philosopher John Locke proposed that human beings are born in a state that he referred to as tabula rasa. What Locke meant was that he believed the human mind at birth is a complete but receptive blank slate upon which experience imprints knowledge. Individual human beings are born with no innate or built-in mental content. In the beginning, human beings are mentally blank, and our entire resource of knowledge is built up gradually from our experiences and sensory perceptions of the outside world.

Many have offered arguments contrary to what Locke believed. But realistically speaking, there has been little evidence to suggest that human beings are born with anything more than a natural ability to learn. Most modern theories of human development have assumed Locke was reasonably accurate in his thesis. Psychoanalytic, behavioral, social learning, and humanistic theories of human development assume that human beings are born with little in terms of innate knowledge, and that all skills needed to survive physically, socially, and emotionally must be learned.

An individual's relative maturity is largely defined in terms of skill development. For example, when a child enters his or her school years, a determination is made as to whether or not that child has developed the skills needed to function in school. Entry into kindergarten is frequently predicated upon whether or not the child has achieved such skills as bladder control, a minimal level of social adaptibility, the ability to listen and follow basic instructions, and other basic skills. If and when a child is denied entry into kindergarten, that determination is generally stated in terms of the child's deficiency in having mastered these basic skills. The child is said to be too immature to succeed in school. Usually when a child is denied entry into kindergarten, he or she is held out of school for one year to acquire the skills needed, or the child is referred to a program designed for that purpose, such as Head Start.

When you examine any individual's progression in life, it is apparent that the hallmarks of his or her level of maturity are defined by the mastery of certain skills. When the individual fails to demonstrate a mastery of age-appropriate skills, the progression is disrupted or halted.

Anyone who has significant time involved in the provision of addiction treatment services has heard this common axiom, "Once a person begins to use alcohol and/or drugs to excess, that person's emotional, social, and intellectual development becomes arrested at that point in time." My observation of addicted individuals would tend to support that conclusion. It truly does appear that when individuals learn to rely on alcohol and/or other mood-altering substances to deal with the challenges of day-to-day living, these individuals cease to advance emotionally and socially. Even if these individuals do acquire new intellectual skills, they seem incapable of applying these skills to resolve or overcome the challenges of life.

According to statistics offered by the Substance Abuse and Mental Health Services Administration (2003), among the groups of individuals who were most frequently identified as being in need of treatment for illicit drug use, the group with the highest representation was those who ranged between the ages of eighteen and twenty-five years (5.7 percent of the total U.S. population). This was followed by individuals who ranged in age from twelve to seventeen years (4.6 percent of the total population). From these estimates we can assume that in most instances, the average age of onset for substance abuse problems is very likely to be somewhere in the teenage and early adulthood years of individual development.

Then, if an individual's development becomes arrested at the onset of the substance abuse, many adults who present for addictions treatment have not matured beyond the level of a teenager. Again, my observations would tend to support such a conclusion. It is not unusual to accurately compare the behavior observed of an adult substance-dependent patient with that of a teenager. Most substance-dependent patients truly can be described as being developmentally immature when compared an average same-age adult. This is why I regard substance abuse problems as being more related to an individual's intellectual, social, and emotional development than to a disease process.

The key to changing the behavior of a substance-abusing patient is to facilitate the acquisition of skills which would allow a more direct and constructive fulfillment of needs. Patients need to learn what to do *instead* of turning to the use of mood-altering chemicals!

To date, the imparting of skills has not been a key element in our society's treatment of substance use disorders. So, why is my assessment of these matters any more accurate than most of that which predates this endeavor? My response to this important question is that all of the empirically sound research conducted recently has demonstrated that alternative treatment approaches, especially skill development, have established efficacy rates well above traditional models.

The most comprehensive and empirically sound study about what is effective in treating substance use disorders is outlined in the *Handbook of Alcoholism Treatment Approaches: Effective Alternatives, Second Edition* (Hester and Miller, 1995). Reid K. Hester and William R. Miller have been actively involved in researching substance abuse treatment since the late 1970s. These authors are among the most eminent researchers in this area of inquiry to the present date. Contributions made therein have been cited in many notable literary and research efforts.

In chapter two of the *Handbook of Alcoholism Treatment Approaches*, the authors summarize their primary conclusions (Miller and Hester, 1980, 1986a, 1986c, 1986b, 1989) as follows: "General conclusions of these reviews were that (1) there are a number of promising treatment approaches supported by efficacy research and (2) current practice reflects little of this knowledge, and instead relies largely on various strategies for which scientific evidence is lacking" (p. 13).

To identify what worked best, Hester and Miller (1995) employed a meta-analytic approach to examine the relative effectiveness of thirty-three treatment modalities. Studies referencing each of the thirty-three treatment modalities were included if they met the following criteria: 1. the study included at least one treatment intended to impact problematic alcohol consumption; 2. the study compared the treatment(s) with a control condition or with any alternative treatments; 3. a proper procedure (e.g., randomization, case control, matching) was used to equate groups prior to treatment; and 4. the study included at least one outcome measure of drinking and/or of alcohol related problems.

The culmination of this effort resulted in a cumulative evidence score (CES) rating which ranged from +239 to -239, with the positive rating indicating demonstrable effectiveness and a negative rating indicating a lack of demonstrable effectiveness. Among the top four rated treatment modalities were brief intervention (CES = +239), social skills training (CES = +128), motivational enhancement (CES = +87), and community reinforcement approach (CES = +80). The worst four modalities included confrontational counseling (CES = -125), psychotherapy (CES = -127), general alcoholism counseling (CES = -214), and educational lectures/films (CES = -239). A surprising outcome to this analysis was that, overall, the most costly treatment modalities were also the least effective, and the most effective were among the least expensive.

Brief intervention, the most effective of the thirty-three modalities, is most frequently an intervention reserved for individuals having only modest problems with alcohol or other substances. Brief intervention is most appropriately utilized when intervening in the substance use problems of individuals not psychologically or physically reliant.

A basic brief intervention scheme often consists of a screening or assessment effort, one or two counseling sessions to discuss appropriate behavioral goals for the patient, and follow-up to determine if the patient followed recommendations or if further intervention might be needed. The therapist's role in this intervention is to offer the patient direction or guidance toward the use of self-help manuals or other forms of bibliotherapy.

Since our concern is with offering appropriate and effective treatment to substance-dependent individuals, we will examine the treatment approach demonstrated to be the most effective for serious alcohol and drug problems. That, according to Hester and Miller's analysis (1995), is coping and social skills training (CSST).

Chapter thirteen of Hester and Miller's book was written by P. M. Monti, D. J. Rohsenow, S. M. Colby, and D. B. Abrams. Based on an impressive array of empirical research outcome studies, they recommended a core set of skill-training modules which should be incorporated into any comprehensive substance abuse treatment effort. There are fourteen recommended skills training modules:

Refusal Skills
Giving Positive Feedback
Giving Criticism
Receiving Criticism about Drinking/Drug Use
Listening Skills
Conversation Skills
Managing Thoughts about Drinking and Coping with Craving
Managing Negative Thinking
Seemingly Irrelevant Decisions
Developing Sober Supports
Conflict Resolution Skills
Nonverbal Communication
Expressing Feelings
Assertiveness Training

As can be seen, the training modules recommended for treatment of substance abusing patients include how to improve upon social/interpersonal skills, management of emotions and negative thinking, and skills related to dealing with environmental contributions to substance use and relapse. The content of the various skill-training modules are relatively self-explanatory. The title of the module is descriptive of the content of each training module. For a more complete description of the practical content of each of these modules, go to chapter thirteen of Hester and Miller's book (pp. 221–241).

This same chapter includes citations of the empirical research that forms the rational basis for the recommendation of specific skill-training modules. In general, the underlying conceptualization is that the substance abusing client "lacks important coping skills for daily living. These deficits can include lack of adequate skills to regulate positive and negative mood states and to cope with social-interpersonal situations, including work, parenting, or marital relationships. Moreover, coping difficulties can be the result of person—environment interactions" (pp. 221–222).

Remember, our short-term goal is that the patient must begin to learn and implement new, more effective, and constructive strategies for dealing with troublesome thoughts and emotions.

Not every patient who might present for treatment needs to be subjected to all skill-training modules as outlined in Hester and Miller's (1995) informative text. An individual's treatment should be designed according to the patient's need and way of relating to the world. Each patient should be offered skill training tailored to correct his or her unique set of deficits. These deficits might relate to the patient's inability to deal with a broad range of problems, such as how to deal with interpersonal, family, work, or spiritual problems, and so on.

In the final analysis, assisting patients in developing skills relating to any aspect of life (interpersonal, family, work, and so on) will help in dealing with troublesome thoughts and feelings. Their perceptions of how well they might be dealing with these areas of their lives either contribute to or detract from their sense of personal competence and self-worth. Inevitably, if patients who perceive they lack the skills necessary to effectively deal with an aspect of life will be confronted by thoughts and emotions which reflect that deficiency. This, in turn, provides an excuse to escape thoughts and emotions through the use of alcohol and/or drugs.

It is important to provide patients with opportunities to test newfound skills while having access to the support of the treatment environment. This is the primary reason that treatment should be attempted from an intensive outpatient treatment setting. Here, patients will only spend three or four hours each day. This provides patients with ample opportunity to test new skills and to share their successes or failures within the confines of a supportive and instructive environment. If patients need further instruction or encouragement, it is available on a daily basis.

Once patients perceive themselves as more competent and better prepared to deal with the challenges of daily living, they will experience fewer and fewer negative or troublesome thoughts and emotions. In essence, patients learn what to do *instead* of attempting to escape or avoid these thoughts and feelings through the use of mood-altering substances.

STG #4. The patient must create a balanced lifestyle.

Up to this point in the treatment, the individual patient has constructively dealt with denial; the patient has made the connections between the experience of troublesome thoughts and feelings and the use of mood-altering chemicals; and the patient has learned new skills needed to deal with life. The next short-term goal for the patient is to begin to balance his or her life.

Patients enter treatment with a wide variety of deficiencies. Common among of these deficiencies is that all too often these patients have defined their personal identities in narrow terms. Most often, these patients will define themselves by only one role in their day-to-day lives. The problem is that these patients generally think they are unable to perform that role competently.

To develop the ability to see oneself as capable of fulfilling a variety of life roles is what is meant by creating balance. Here is a common example: when you ask any adult to tell you who he or she is, frequently that adult will offer a job title or a job description. Beyond that, it is not uncommon that any individual will appear to be at a loss to say more.

In psychological terms, this means that the individual's self perceptions and self-esteem are entirely dependent upon the perception of how a singular role is fulfilled. This is a very narrow and inadequate means of forming a personal identity. Unfortunately, this is all too common in modern society. Equally unfortunate is that no matter what stage of development we are examining, it appears more and more that individuals attempt to define themselves in terms of singular roles that that they be attempting to fulfill. For example, a teenage boy might only define himself either as a good football player or as an accomplished student. If he does not see himself as moderately successful in comparison to his peers, it is likely that this boy will suffer from distortions of self-perception and low self-esteem.

Self-esteem. Now there's a term we hear frequently, especially with reference to substance use problems and in the subsequent treatment thereof. What does this mean, and why does it seem that everyone should possess high self-esteem?

Self-esteem is, essentially, the way we feel about ourselves, or the extent to which we value or admire ourselves. It is the sense of personal worth we associate with our self-concept (Atwater, 1983). How important is self-esteem in the treatment of addictive disorders? It is certain that an individual's self-concept is a subjective factor that can play a determining role in the development of substance-abusing behavior. If the individual cannot develop a way of seeing themselves as being acceptable, competent, lovable, and worthy of dignity and respect, then troublesome thoughts and feelings will inevitably be experienced. One of the primary reasons that an individual learns to rely on mood-altering substances is to escape from troublesome thoughts and feelings.

That there exists a connection between low self-esteem and substance abuse is well established. Jerome Levin, in his book entitled *Treatment of Alcoholism and Other Addictions* (1987), stated, "All alcoholics suffer from near zero self-esteem. Most of their bluster and reactive grandiosity is a cover for and denial of their abysmally low self-regard." More recently, Taylor, Lloyd, and Warhiedt (2006) conducted an empirical effort to determine whether low self-esteem observed in youth predicted future substance abuse. The study examined whether early reports of self-derogation and peer approval of substance use prospectively predicted drug dependence. Data from three waves of a nine-year prospective study were employed to examine these relationships among a multiethnic sample of 872 young adult males. The author's analysis confirmed that self-derogation and peer approval of substance use independently predicted drug dependence even when early substance use was controlled. John Taylor, one of the authors of this study, commented, "Low self-esteem is kind of a spark plug for self-destructive behavior, and drug use is one of these. It's a fundamental need to have a good sense of self. Without it, people may become pathologically unhappy with themselves, and that can lead to some very serious problems."

There can be little argument as to whether or not self-esteem should be considered to be an important concept in the treatment of addiction. Actually, we all understand that developing positive self-esteem is important, not only to substance-abusing individuals, but to all human beings. The question is, then, how do we get positive self-esteem?

Self-esteem comes from one major source. That source is task mastery. Tasks can only be mastered through practice. The more tasks we are able to master, the more competent we become. The more competent we become, the more we admire and value ourselves. The more we admire and value ourselves, the more we see ourselves as being worthy of acceptance, love, and approval from others. The more we begin to see ourselves as being acceptable, lovable and valued by others, the less vulnerable we become to thoughts and feelings of anger, fear, frustration, and depression.

What tasks are we talking about and what does it take to master these tasks?

In psychology, when a reference is made to the mastering of tasks, we are talking about an individual's ability to demonstrate the acquisition of skills needed to reach a developmental milestone. Once an individual has mastered a specific life task signaling the achievement of a given developmental milestone, the individual is then able to move on to the next indicator of personal growth and development.

Developmental psychology has offered us many theories offering ways of understanding how individuals grow and develop. Regardless of a given theory's developmental focus, human development is most often described in terms of an individual's ability to master specific tasks.

According to Freud's theory (1905), an individual has to successfully pass through five psychosexual stages of development in order to develop into a normal adult. If the requirements of any given developmental stage are not met, the individual becomes fixated at that stage and is unable to continue normal development until the fixation is resolved. Passage through the first three stages, the oral, anal, and phallic stages, involves receiving or acquiring physical satisfaction and is centered on the erogenous zones. Normal passage through these stages occurs from birth to approximately six years of age. Completion of the latency stage, age six to puberty, involves the successful acquisition of cultural and social skills. Completion of the last stage, the genital stage, rests on the successful balancing of heterosexual desires. Freud also postulated that normal development depended on the successful resolution of the Oedipus complex for males and the Electra complex for females. According to Freud's theory, certain tasks must be mastered in order for a child to develop into a normal adult.

No matter what developmental theory one might choose to examine, normal human development is marked by the individual's demonstration that specific life tasks have been mastered. For Piaget (1967), a child's cognitive development is marked by the ability to acquire specific cognitive abilities which are demonstrated behaviorally.

According to Erik Erikson (1963), an individual must progress through eight psychosocial stages from infancy through later adulthood. Successful passage through each of Erickson's developmental stages is marked by successful resolution of specific opposing conflicts. Resolution of these conflicts requires the individual to, through observable actions, demonstrate that he or she has acquired specific skills and abilities appropriate to each stage of development.

All perspectives regarding human development assert that individuals must be able to master certain life tasks in order to develop into normal, fully functioning adults.

Alfred Adler's theory of personality is useful when relating an individual's growth and development to the exhibition of abnormal behavior (Corey, 1985; Dworetzky, 1982; and Gilliland, James, Roberts, and Bowman, 1894), such as alcohol and drug abuse. It is believed that Alder formulated his theories based upon his own individual development. Adler endured a rather miserable childhood marked by illness, accidents, and failures in school. The negative impact of these experiences contributed to a relentless drive to rid himself of feelings of inferiority and to strive toward superiority. Hence came the term "inferiority complex."

According to Adler, whatever meaning life has for an individual depends upon how the individual faces up to the tests that life presents. The ultimate indicator of how well an individual faces up to life's tests is the extent of willingness to take risks—courage. However, human beings are social beings, and their behavior is understood only in terms of the social meaning.

Social meaning, as defined by Adler, means "wanting to belong." Whether this belonging is in terms of family, significant others, social groups, professions, etc., the goal of belonging is embedded in life tasks. According to Adler's theory, there are five major life tasks that are presented to each person. These tasks are:

1. *Society*—Life tasks with regard to society are geared toward developing a sense of responsibility to humankind and the environment;
2. *Occupation*—To survive as a society, we must learn to cooperate. Individuals must develop a willingness to assume an occupational role and must learn to gain satisfaction from that role;
3. *Sex*—Developing an understanding of and an ability to relate to the opposite sex;
4. *Spirituality*—Coming to an understanding of the existence and nature of God and developing a spiritual identity;
5. *"I" and "Me"*—Developing an understanding of the individual self, the "I" as the subjective self, and the "me" as the objective self.

All life tasks are socially embedded. Social interest is part of the individual's psychological equipment to be used in striving for perfection.

When I work with substance-using patients, I have generally utilized Adler's life tasks as a way of explaining what I mean when I tell the patient to develop a balanced lifestyle. Essentially, the treatment approaches I have utilized represent a means to guide the patient toward the development of basic competencies to assist the individual to accomplish these life tasks. The more capable the patient becomes, the more the patient believes that he or she has value and is worthy of admiration. Simply, the patient builds self-esteem through the mastery of life's tasks.

Adler coined the term inferiority complex. According to Adler, all abnormal behavior stems from the discouragement resulting from the inferiority complex. There are five components to the inferiority complex:

1. An individual has a mistaken opinion of himself or herself and the world. That is, the person has a mistaken style of life guided by the adoption of mistaken goals;
2. The individual will resort to abnormal behavior aimed at safeguarding that self opinion;
3. Such safeguarding occurs when the individual is confronted with situations which will probably be met unsuccessfully;
4. The mistake consists of being self-centered rather than taking humankind into consideration;
5. The individual is not consciously aware of these processes.

The person with an inferiority complex seeks escape from an unbearable situation by a compensatory move toward superiority. This move, however, is not aimed at problem-solving, but rather it is aimed at safeguarding his or her opinion of self. The maladjusted person vacillates between feeling inferior and superior and is highly ambitious, but lacks the courage to take necessary risks. Avoidance, displacement, denial, projection, etc., are used to save the individual from the ultimate threat—being seen as inferior.

Obviously, the individual who feels inferior lacks self esteem. Such an individual will engage in behaviors designed to preserve whatever remains of an ailing self-concept. Sometimes, the individual attempts to compensate for these feelings through the use of alcohol and other mood-altering chemicals to create the illusion or sense of being superior.

This accurately describes what is seen in any individual that might present for treatment of substance use disorders. When sober, such an individual appears to engage in a great deal of self-loathing.

Individuals entering treatment are frequently extremely self-centered and appear to be incapable of seeing the world as it really is. These individuals greatly fear how others might see them because they feel inferior to others. They attempt to save themselves by exhibiting defense mechanisms such as avoidance, displacement, denial, projection, etc.

When the feelings of inferiority can no longer be tolerated, a substance-abusing individual attempts to escape by using a mood-altering substance. The substance creates the illusion that the individual is superior. Thus, while under the influence of the mood-altering chemical, that individual will exhibit a façade of grandiosity.

Vacillation between self loathing and grandiosity—is this not what we observe of the patients we see entering treatment for addictions? I believe it is.

The only way to move away from feeling inferior and overcome a lack of self-esteem is to strive for superiority. This striving must be directed toward the mastery of life tasks such as those described by Adler and others. It is not sufficient to develop competencies relative to the fulfillment of a singular role in life. The individual recovering from substance use disorder must strive to master tasks relating to interactions with others as well as with the environment. The individual must develop a willingness to assume a constructive occupational role in life, an ability to relate to the opposite sex, and an understanding of the existence of God. The individual must begin to understand him or herself, both subjectively and objectively. Only by mastering tasks related to such a range of roles will the individual feel competent, capable, and worthy of love and admiration. Only through this type of striving can the individual develop balance in life.

Now, as Adler was very careful to point out, superiority is a fictional goal. None of us can become perfect. All that any individual can do is to gradually and progressively attempt to approximate the idea of perfection or superiority. The closer that an individual comes to approximating this idea, or fictional goal, the more the individual becomes insulated from feelings of inferiority. The patient develops realistic self-esteem by way of task mastery over a broad range of life tasks.

It should be obvious that such an undertaking is lifelong. An individual patient will not likely achieve a balanced lifestyle or be rid of all feelings of inferiority while in treatment. All that a treatment professional can do is to start the patient on his or her quest toward developing a more balanced lifestyle by pointing out that the individual patient must attempt to become competent in a variety of roles.

As treatment professionals, it is our responsibility to encourage the recovering individual to begin this life quest. It is a quest toward achieving balance in life and toward enabling the patient to realistically see him or herself as being competent and valuable. It really doesn't matter what perspective a given treatment provider might adhere to or how this challenge is presented. It is vitally important to make the treatment relevant to the needs of the individual patient. I have used Adler's theory to exemplify one way of accomplishing this goal. This perspective and way of approaching the attainment of this short-term goal has worked for me with many patients. It is not the only perspective nor is it the only approach that can be applied to assist a patient in attaining this last treatment goal. It is just one among many perspectives that can be utilized in a comprehensive treatment plan.

In this chapter, I have outlined four short-term goals essential in any comprehensive effort to treat substance use disorders. No individual patient can successfully enter into recovery from a substance use disorder until he or she has successfully attained or closely approximated these four goals. Once an individual has attained the short-term goals described in this chapter, that individual will be much more prepared to deal with life without resorting to the use of alcohol or other drugs than any patient subjected only to traditional twelve-step treatment. To date, the existing research supports this.

References

Chapter Thirteen

Atwater, E. (1983). *Psychology or Adjustment, Second Edition.* (pp. 113–130).

Englewood Cliffs, NJ: Prentice-Hall, Inc.

Corey, G. (1985). *Theory and Practice of Group Counseling.* Belmont, CA: Brooks/Cole Publishing Co.

Dworetzky, J. P. (1982). *Psychology.* St. Paul, MN: West Publishing Co.

Erikson, E. H. (1963). *Childhood and Society.* New York, NY: Norton.

Freud, S. (1905). Three essays on sexuality. J. Strachey (Ed.), *The Standard Edition of the Complete Psychological Works (Vol. 7).* London, UK: Hogarth Press. (originally published, 1905).

Gilliland, B. E., James, R. K., Roberts, G. T., and Bowman, J. T. (1984). *Theories and Strategies in Counseling and Psychotherapy.* Englewood Cliffs, NJ: Prentice-Hall, Inc.

Hazelden (1975). *Dealing with denial.* Center City, MN: Hazelden Community Services.

Hester, R., and Miller, W. (1995). What Works? *Handbook of Alcoholism Treatment Approaches: Effective Alternatives.* Boston, MA: Allyn and Bacon.

Levin, J. D. (1987). *Treatment of Alcoholism and Other Addictions: A self-Psychology Approach* (p. 292). Northvale, NJ: Jason Aaronson, Inc.

Lieberman, M. A., Yalom, I. D., and Miles, M. B. (1973). *Encounter groups: First facts.* New York, NY: Basic Books.

Locke, J. (1690). *An Essay Concerning Human Understanding.* K. P. Winkler (Ed.), (pp. 33–36) Indianapolis, IN: Hackett Publishing Company.

MacDonough, T. S. (1976). Evaluation of the effectiveness of intensive confrontation in changing the behavior of alcohol and drug abusers. *Behavior Therapy*, **24**, 461–504.

Miller, W., and Hester, R. K. (1980). Treating problem drinkers: Modern approaches. W. R. Miller (Ed.), *The Addictive Behaviors: Treatment of Alcoholism, Drug Abuse, Smoking, and Obesity* (pp. 11–141). Oxford, UK: Pergamon Press.

Miller W., and Hester, R. K. (1986a). The effectiveness of alcoholism treatment methods: what research reveals. W.R. Miller and N. Heather (Eds.), *Treating Addictive Behaviors: Process of Change* (pp. 121–174). New York, NY: Plenum Press.

Miller, W., and Hester, R. K. (1986b). Inpatient alcoholism treatment: Who benefits? *American Psychologist*, **41**, 794–805.

Miller, W., and Hester, R. K. (1986c). Matching problem drinkers with optimal treatments. W. R. Miller and N. Heather (Eds.), *Treating Addictive Behaviors: Process of Change* (pp. 175–203). New York, NY: Plenum Press.

Miller, W., and Hester, R. K. (1989). Inpatient alcoholism treatment: rules of evidence and burden of proof. *American Psychologist*, **44**, 1245–1246.

Miller, W. R., Benefield, R. G., and Tonigan, J. S. (1993). Enhancing motivation for change in problem drinking: A controlled comparison of two therapist's styles. *Journal of Consulting and Clinical Psychology*, **61**, 455–461.

Pavlov, I. P. (1927). *Conditioned reflexes*. New York, NY: Oxford University Press.

Piaget, J., and Inhelder, B. (1967). *The Psychology of the Child*. (H. Weaver, trans.). New York, NY: Basic Books.

Rogers, C. A. (1959). A theory of therapy, personality, and interpersonal relationships as developed in the client-centered framework. Reprinted in H. Kirshenbaum and V. Henderson (Eds.) *The Carl Rogers Reader* (1989). Boston, MA: Houghton Mifflin.

Substance Abuse and Mental Health Services Administration (2003). National Survey of Substance Abuse Treatment Services (N-SSATS) 2003. Web site: http://www. oas.samhsa.gov/2k3/ NSSATS/NSSATS.pdf.

Taylor, J., Lloyd, D. A., and Warheit, G. J. (2006). Self-derogation, peer factors, and drug dependence among a multiethnic sample of young adults. *Journal of Child and Adolescent Substance Abuse,* **15(2)**, 39–51.

Watson, J. B. (1929). *Psychology from the standpoint of a behaviorist*, 3rd Ed. Philadelphia, PA: Lippincott.

Webster's II New Riverside Dictionary. (1984). (p. 457). Boston, MA: Houghton Mifflin Company.

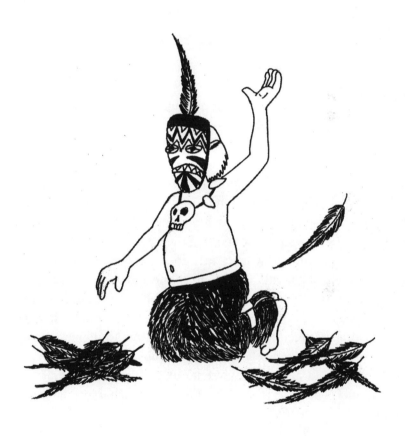

Chapter 14

Treatment Perspective and Technique

In the previous chapter, I thoroughly outlined a set of four short-term treatment goals which the substance-using patient must achieve to have a reasonable chance for freedom from a reliance upon alcohol and/or drugs. As much as possible, I outlined only *what* must be accomplished. I have not yet provided any clear guidance as to useful techniques. I will now offer more specific guidance as to which therapeutic perspectives and techniques might be most effective in assisting patients to achieve the short-term goals.

First, I must address what clearly does not work in the treatment of substance-reliant patients. The number one approach to eliminate due to its proven ineffectiveness is the traditional twelve-step treatment model. The next in line for elimination as an effective therapeutic technique is any technique from a perspective to which the patient cannot relate to. It is entirely useless to employ any treatment approach which has no relevance to the patient's existing problems, the patient's current and past experiences, or the patient's characteristic way of relating to the objective world.

It is absolutely essential for the therapist to match the choice therapeutic perspective and technique to the patient's needs and way of relating to the world. Every therapist knows that in all therapeutic efforts, regardless of the problem a patient might exhibit, the choice of theoretical perspective and technique depends upon the patient, not the therapist's preference. For example, sometimes therapists refer to themselves as being behaviorists, psychoanalysts, or cognitive therapists. This therapist has only a minimal chance of being helpful to you because this therapist desires to approach all problems from a solitary perspective.

Take a moment to think about this concept. Let us use an analogy from practical day-to-day life. Would you allow a mechanic whose only tool consists of a five-inch crescent wrench to attempt to repair your 2006 BMW Z4? Now a five-inch crescent wrench is a good tool for a mechanic to possess. Nevertheless, it is just one tool and it is not well suited for all mechanical tasks. If you were to allow this mechanic to attempt to repair your BMW, you might get lucky and your prized vehicle's problems might get fixed with just this wrench. However, the chances to successfully repair your vehicle increase substantially if you assume that your mechanic might need more than one tool to fix all problems. The same is true of personal problems.

Previously, I stated that there is no singular way to treat depression. I will again use the problem of depression to exemplify my point. If a patient presents with symptoms of depression, what course of treatment do I recommend? Do I refer the patient to a physician or a psychiatrist so the patient can be prescribed antidepressant medication? Do I choose to treat the patient alone by providing cognitive behavioral therapy? Do I choose psychoanalysis? Rational-emotive therapy? Gestalt therapy? Which approach is best? Well, if I only know one perspective, my choice is simple. However, my chances for being successful in helping the patient are limited.

Depression is different in every person. What might be an effective approach in treating one person might be totally useless for another. Actually, it would be marvelous if depression was the same for all persons. We could eliminate depression as a problem for everyone very quickly and easily if that were the case. Unfortunately, this is not the case for depression. Similarly, it is also not the case for substance use disorders either.

This tendency toward over-generalization has been my biggest protest regarding the continual reliance upon traditional twelve-step as the only means of treating substance use disorders. Twelve-step treatment offers only one approach to treating substance use problems. At its very foundation is the basic assumption that all individuals suffering from substance use disorders have a singular disease and there is only one way to treat it. This is nonsense.

Like depression, every patient who presents for treatment of a substance use disorder comes with a unique set of problems to be addressed. Additionally, every substance-reliant patient comes to treatment with a unique way of understanding, relating to, and interacting with the objective world. As such, there can be no singular theoretical perspective which completely explains how and why substance use problems occur. Nor is there a singular set of techniques that can be utilized to treat all substance-reliant patients.

It is of great importance to come to an operational conceptualization of the individual patient's problems. Forming an operational conceptualization of the patient's problem is undertaken for more than the sole purpose of diagnosis. By gaining as much current and historical information as possible about a patient, not only does it become easier to accurately diagnose or pinpoint specific problems or problem areas, but what actually emerges from this holistic collection of data is a mapping of the individual's path in life up to the current time. This map illustrates the major experiences that influenced the individual's physical, personal, intellectual, social, and moral development. This is a map that can also allow the clinician to understand and appreciate how this individual views the self, relates to others, and to his or her environment.

The image such a map can provide for a clinician can be extremely valuable in making preliminary decisions about perspective and the set of therapeutic techniques most relevant to the needs of the patient. By coming to a holistic understanding of an individual patient, the clinician can make choices regarding which theoretical perspective can most accurately explain what is illustrated in the patient's set of major life experiences and how that patient has come to view, think, feel, and behave.

Imagine that your patient has learned to rely heavily on intellectual abilities to understand the world. This particular patient attempts to relate to the world through the use of logic and rationality. Now, if the clinician begins to discuss this patient's problems in terms of how the patient *feels* about his or her interactions with others or how the patient *feels* about how he or she experiences the world, the patient's response to this approach is going to be one of puzzlement and confusion. This is a patient that talks about what his or her thoughts are, and whether or not what he or she is experiencing makes any rational or logical sense. This is a person who attempts to resolve most problems intellectually.

As one might imagine, the best way a clinician can begin to align with the intellectual patient is by approaching this particular patient through the application of a perspective emphasizing cognition as a means of relating to the world. Appropriate perspectives from which a clinician might approach this particular patient might include cognitive therapy, cognitive/behavioral therapy, or rational emotive therapy. Such approaches as these match the patient's way of relating to world.

Conversely, if your patient relates to world in terms of emotions, approaching the patient's problem(s) through the application of one of the cognitive perspectives is likely to be meaningless. The feeling patient is less concerned about thoughts than how interactions with the objective world make him or her feel. Emotional response is the focus, not whether or not the patient is experiencing the world in rational or logical ways. As such, approaches which address emotions are appropriate for this particular patient. Appropriate perspectives most helpful might include client-centered therapy, gestalt, or even psychoanalytic/psychodynamic therapies.

Likewise, the impulsive patient might best be approached through the application of any of the behavioral perspectives.

In other words, if the objectives are to develop a relationship with a patient to engender trust and to use techniques relevant to the patient's world view, then the clinician is responsible for initiating that relationship by adopting an appropriate perspective. The therapist must attempt to match the approach to the needs of the patient in order to be perceived as empathic.

This attempt on the part of any treatment provider has historically been referred to as *patient-treatment matching*. Experienced, competently trained, effective therapists routinely match their approach to treatment with the needs of the patient. Such treatment providers do not employ the "one tool conquers all problems" approach.

Unfortunately, no such thing can be said of addictions treatment in the United States. More than 90 percent of all the addictions treatment programs in our nation rely primarily on the traditional twelve-step treatment approach (Roman and Blum, 1997). This traditional approach represents the epitome of a "one tool fixes all problems" mentality. The outcomes that have been demonstrated utilizing this approach have been miserable—no better than no treatment at all.

There has been no widespread attempt to employ a strict application of treatment matching within the addictions treatment industry in our country. In recent years, however, there have been a few experimental efforts that have loosely attempted to employ the concept of treatment matching to the treatment of substance use disorders.

The most notable of these attempts to match treatment to the needs of the patients was called Project Match (Project Match Research Group, 1993). Funded by the National Institute on Alcohol Abuse and Alcoholism (NIAAA), Project Match was undertaken with an assumption that no single treatment approach is effective for all alcoholics. It was hypothesized that a more promising strategy might be to assign patients to alternative treatments based on the specific needs and the characteristics of the patients.

In Project Match, two independent but parallel matching studies were conducted. One of the studies included participants recruited from outpatient treatment settings. The other involved participants recruited from outpatient aftercare who had received inpatient treatment for alcoholism. Approximately 1,500 patients volunteered to serve as subjects in this study. These volunteer subjects were randomly assigned to one of three treatment groups: twelve-step facilitation therapy (TSF); cognitive-behavioral coping skills (CBCS); or motivational enhancement therapy (MET). Follow-ups were conducted at three-month intervals for one year after completion of the twelve-week treatment period, and subjects were evaluated for changes in drinking patterns, functional status/quality of life, and treatment services utilization. The interaction effects with selected patient characteristics were also studied.

The TSF delivered in this experiment relied on the premise that alcoholism is a spiritual and medical disease, with the primary objectives of fostering an acceptance of the disease of alcoholism and developing a commitment to attend Alcoholics Anonymous (AA) and to work on the Twelve Steps of AA (Miller and Rollnick, 2002). The research group was careful to point out that TSF was not intended to be a test of AA as a treatment per se, but it was designed to encourage the subjects' involvement in AA.

The CBCS was based on social learning theory which regards drinking behavior to be related to problems in the individual's life. Emphasis was placed on overcoming skills deficits and increasing skills to help the individual cope with situations believed to precipitate relapse (Project Match Research Group, 1997).

The MET was based on the principles of motivational interviewing (Mattson, 1994). This treatment was intended to build patient motivation for change and to foster a commitment to change.

The primary objective of this study was to determine whether various groups responded differently to treatments. However, subjects were *randomly* assigned to one of the three treatment conditions. Then, subjects were evaluated with regard to ten attributes which the study group referred to as matching variables. These variables were: 1) severity of alcohol involvement, 2) cognitive impairment, 3) client conceptual level, 4) gender, 5) meaning seeking, 6) motivational readiness to change, 7) psychiatric severity, 8) social support, 9) sociopathy, and 10) alcohol typology. Measures for each of these ten variables were selected, consisting of various interviews and testing instruments, and it was anticipated that interactions would be observed as outlined by sixteen hypothesized contrasts (Project Research Group, 1997).

Each of the three manual-guided treatments was delivered over a period of twelve weeks, one session per week. The exception to this was that the MET treatment was delivered in four sessions which took place on the first, second, sixth, and twelfth weeks of the study. Each treatment was delivered on an individual basis by therapists that were specifically trained to deliver the respective treatments in a uniform and consistent manner. All of the therapy sessions were videotaped, and 25 percent of these sessions were selected for monitoring by supervisors to ensure that the various treatments were conducted as intended. The primary outcome measures consisted of percent of days abstinent (PDA) and the number of drinks per drinking day (DDD).

Project Match was estimated to have cost more than twenty-seven million dollars and was conducted over a period of eight years. Well, what did this eight-year, twenty-seven-million-dollar effort end up revealing? As unfortunate as it may seem, not much of anything!

The good news was that there was a substantial improvement in the amount of PDA and DDD of drinking for both the outpatient and aftercare subjects from the baseline measurement (before treatment) and to each of the follow-up points designated in the study. The study mentioned that there was a slight deterioration on these measures at one-year post-treatment. The only treatment by attribute interaction observed was that subjects who were assigned to the TSF outpatient group who also exhibited less severe psychiatric symptoms had statistically more abstinent days that did those who had been assigned to the CBCS outpatient group. The difference was an average of four more days of abstinence for those who participated in the TSF group compared to the CBCS group.

There were also two effects observed that were not originally hypothesized. Subjects who appeared to have higher motivation had significantly better outcomes. Additionally, subjects who appeared to have greater social support for drinking evidenced worse outcomes across all treatment conditions.

The bad news is that little else could be gleaned from this incredibly expensive and complex research effort.

Now, let us examine this study to determine if we can find some reasons why such an expansive effort yielded so little.

First, let's look at the treatment approaches utilized in this study. Do you see something that is obviously missing here? *There was no control group!* What was the point in comparing three treatment conditions if no comparison to a "no treatment" group could be made? What we really do not know is whether or not any of these treatment conditions yielded better outcomes than no treatment at all.

After NIAAA director, Enoch Gordis, MD (1997), received an abundance of critical comments regarding the interpretation of the outcomes of Project Match, he offered the following comments:

After the findings from Project Match were publicized, it appeared clear from the comments received by NIAAA that these findings, in some instances, had been misinterpreted. Therefore, I believe it is useful to clarify again what Project Match was and what it was not. Project Match was a study of patient-treatment matching; it was not a study of treatment efficacy. While it was heartening to learn that patients who participated in all three treatment arms did well, this study was not to test whether treatment (versus no treatment) works but whether patients, based on their characteristics, responded better to one therapy versus another.

Then why bother to include treatment modality as a variable? Would it not make as much sense to simply assign patients to a single treatment modality according to the patients' characteristics and compare that to a similar set of patients in a no-treatment comparison group? Oh, that's right; that had already been done, repeatedly. What is the point of attempting to determine if patients, based on their characteristics, responded differently to various treatment modalities if it could not be determined whether or not any of these treatments offered anything above no treatment at all?

Now, let us look as what Project Match termed "patient characteristics." Can we accurately assume that the ten attributes selected to represent patient characteristics in Project MATCH actually represent the individual characteristics of any of the patients? I guess we can say that gender could be assumed to be an individual characteristic. Perhaps, even sociopathy could be considered to be descriptive of a set of individual characteristics. However, I really do not see how the remaining variables which this project refers to as "characteristics" are really that at all. For example, would not "social support" more accurately be considered an environmental influence as opposed to an individual characteristic? Does it not seem that severity of alcohol involvement and alcohol typology are somewhat redundant, since typology is, in many respects, tied to severity of involvement? Both of these latter variables appeared to be rather ill-defined, and are likely interrelated.

The remaining characteristics (cognitive impairment, client conceptual level, meaning seeking, motivational readiness to change, and psychiatric severity) that were identified as variable characteristics in this project are not individual characteristics at all. These are better defined as behavioral manifestations that may, or may not, be a reflection of any set of individual characteristics. For example, are all individuals who exhibit a certain degree of any psychiatric problem all characteristically similar? Maybe these psychiatrically impaired individuals are similar depending upon whether or not we would be making reference to a specific psychiatric disorder. But that was not what was done in this project. It made reference to severity of problems across a broad range of disorders. There could be no assumption, according to the definition of this variable, that patients were characteristically or psychologically similar in any way.

As can be seen, Project Match suffered from some serious conceptual problems before it was implemented. It offered no real comparison of treatment modality. It attempted to define individual characteristics very loosely, to say the least. Then, most alarmingly, subjects were randomly assigned to the three treatment modalities in both arms of the project. Project Match made no actual attempt to match anybody to any treatment. No wonder there were no real results.

There were many, many other problems with this insanely expensive and lengthy attempt to simulate real research as well. In his review of Project Match, Bufe (1998) outlines several major biasing factors that certainly appeared to influence the outcome of this study. Bufe's review outlines how the subject selection processes, patients' expectations, and the manner in which the treatments utilized in the study were structured and delivered served to bias the outcome of the study. Bufe summarized his review by stating, "But there does seem to one clear lesson in Project Match: if you introduce enough positive biasing factors, almost any form of treatment will 'produce' a positive outcome."

When the time is taken to carefully look at how Project Match was designed, and look all the various ways that bias was introduced into design of the project, it makes one wonder what exactly this study was intended to accomplish. After all, the Project Match Research Group included two NIAAA coordinators, four coordinating center staff, fifteen clinical research unit staff, eight collaborating investigators, and five individuals serving as a data monitoring board, all of whom had doctoral degrees or medical degrees. Additionally, there were also eighty specially trained psychotherapists who delivered the various treatments at the twenty collaborating facilities (Project Research Group, 1997). In all, there were 130 highly trained clinical professionals who were involved in administration, treatment, and analysis of this project. With this much expertise on hand, it should have been easy for those in charge of the design of this project to eliminate the bias and lack of control inherent in this project's design. Perhaps this project was intended to produce the exact outcomes that resulted.

One of the primary conclusions voiced by the investigators involved in this project was that "the lack of robust matching effects suggests that providers need not consider client characteristics considered in Project Match when assigning patients to treatment" (Project Match Research Group, 1997). As far as these NIAAA supported investigators were concerned, the notion that patient–treatment matching could result in better outcomes was completely invalid. They appeared to believe there is no need to offer further consideration to this possibility. Remember, Project Match was funded by the NIAAA which maintains a close alliance with the National Council on Alcoholism and Drug Dependence (NCADD). The NCADD has vehemently supported the disease concept of addiction. Additionally, the NCADD has served as the public face for Alcoholics Anonymous and the twelve-step treatment industry.

Could it be that the intent behind Project Match was simply to maintain the status quo within our nation's existing treatment industry? I do believe that there is sufficient evidence to suggest the possible existence of such intent. Others have voiced this sentiment as well. Stanton Peele (1998) offered these comments in summary of his review of Project Match.

Project Match represents a massive effort to shoehorn a large amorphous peg into a small square hole. That it fails in this impossible task does not bother the health-care industry, however. This is because, whether or not it accounts for the behavior of alcoholics, the medicalization of alcoholism succeeds in justifying the mission and policies of government and treatment agencies and professionals.

Considering the financial resources allocated to Project Match, and the expertise made available to steer this project, it seems almost unthinkable that the research design and methodology employed in this effort could be as deplorable as it was without such intent. I would suggest that Project Match was just another attempt at misdirection—which seems to have become typical of those who have a vested interest in maintaining the status quo in our nation's treatment industry.

Although patient–treatment matching is still advocated by some in this nation, and there continues to be interest in this notion in terms of research, Project Match appeared to do as I believe it was intended. It put the brakes, at least temporarily, on the notion that patient–treatment matching be considered the "cutting edge" in the addictions treatment field. This effect was substantially achieved despite the fact that Project Match provided no test of this hypothesis at all.

Since the results of Project Match have become common knowledge, attempts to demonstrate that patient-treatment matching might be a viable approach have become few. This is probably due to the fact that the NIAAA and other factions interested in maintaining the status quo have latched on to the notion there is no need to consider this possibility. As such, funds available to support further research into the concept of patient-treatment matching in the addictions field have become very limited. Still, a few efforts continue to demonstrate treatment matching can result in better outcome in the treatment of addictions.

For example, in an attempt to demonstrate that alcohol treatments should be tailored to address the multi-dimensional needs of the individual, researchers Franzke, Clifford, and Maisto (2001) from New York University utilized data collected as part of a larger NIAAA-funded alcohol treatment outcome study to demonstrate that matching subjects to specific treatment modalities on the basis of the subjects' level of social functioning could result in better treatment outcomes. The authors suggested that subjects who suffer from alcohol-related problems often experience difficulties in social functioning. As such, poor social functioning might contribute to problematic drinking.

A treatment-matching hypothesis was tested regarding the levels of social functioning and the type of treatment (i.e., community reinforcement approach or cognitive behavioral). The statistical analysis of the effort revealed that patients who were correctly matched to treatment were drinking significantly fewer drinks per day, relative to patients who had been incorrectly matched.

Other studies have attempted to match patient to treatments on the basis of the severity of the patients' problems to the level of treatment intensity (Timko and Sempel, 2004). These authors, not surprisingly, found that dual diagnosis patients who exhibited severe symptoms benefited significantly from their involvement in high-intensity treatment programs. It was interesting to note that the authors defined high intensity treatment programs as those which offered the following treatment services: detoxification, self-help groups, available psychiatrists and psychologists on staff, psychopharmacology, couples/family counseling, pyschoeducation for patients, pyschoeducation for families, religious counseling, peer counseling, daily living skills training, social skills training, vocational counseling, work therapy, occupational therapy, exercise, organized recreation, films and movies, social hours, and clubs.

In recent times, there have also been a number of studies that have examined patient relapse in relation to certain personality characteristics and to problems such as depression and anxiety. While these studies were not attempts to match patients to specific treatments based on either personality characteristics or mental problems, the results of many of these studies do have strong implications for patient-treatment matching.

For example, one European study examined the relationship between depression and anxiety in patients and their subsequent relapse (Willinger, et al., 2002). In this study 521 patients with a DSM III-R diagnosis of alcohol dependence without major depressive disorder took part in a European multi-center study. The object of the study was to evaluate the impact of mood, affect, and personality on predicting relapse to uncontrolled drinking during a one-year treatment study. Depressive symptoms were assessed using the Hamilton Depression Scale (Hamilton, 1960). Anxiety was assessed using the State-Trait Anxiety Inventory (Speilberger and Gorsuch, 1983). Personality traits were measured by the Tridimensional Personality Questionnaire (Cloninger, 1987). The results of the study indicated that anxiety as a stable trait, and personality traits such as high novelty-seeking and low harm-avoidance—covering exploratory excitability, impulsiveness, disorderliness, and uninhibited optimism—predicted relapse. The authors concluded that the measures utilized in their study could have direct clinical application for predicting relapse to uncontrolled drinking in both male and female detoxified alcohol-dependent patients. Also stated was the conclusion that the findings indicated the importance of additional therapeutic treatment.

An earlier study (Janowski, et al., 1999) attempted to evaluate the role of personality in the short-term outcome of alcohol/substance use disorder patients. In this study, detoxifying alcohol/substance use disorder patients were administered the Myers-Briggs Type Indicator (MBTI) (Myers et al., 1998), the Tridimensional Personality Questionnaire (TPQ) (Cloninger, 1987)), the Michigan Alcoholism Screening Test (MAST) (Selzer, 1971), the CAGE Questionnaire (Ewing, 1984), and the Beck Depression Inventory (BDI) (Beck, 1996). These patients were then evaluated over a period of one month for relapse and attendance at self-help group meetings. Results of the study indicated that high TPQ persistence scale scores predicted abstinence. When thinking and feeling groups (as indicated by MBTI) were considered both separately and in combination, high scores predicted abstinence. High TPQ persistence scale scores and low shyness with strangers and fear of uncertainty subscale scores predicted attendance at self-help group meetings. High MBTI extroversion and high MBTI thinking scores also predicted attendance at self-help group meetings. When the extroverted and introverted types and the thinking and feeling types respectively were combined, as with abstinence, high scores predicted attendance at self-help group meetings. Age, gender, CAGE, MAST, and BDI scores did not predict outcome. The authors of this piece concluded that specific personality variables may predict abstinence and attendance at self-help group meetings in recently detoxified alcoholics, and that this may have prognostic and therapeutic significance.

While the research effort just cited was small in scale (only sixty-two subjects), the results confirmed outcomes from other studies, which examined the relationship between personality as defined by the TPQ and relapse. For example, Sellman et al. (1997) found that alcoholics who relapsed had, on average, lower TPQ persistence scale scores.

The Myers-Briggs Type Indicator has not been widely utilized in addictions treatment (Meyers and McCaulley, 1985). However, previous research efforts have suggested that being introverted and having an external locus of control have generally been found to predict a poor prognosis (Tarnai and Young, 1983; Canton et al., 1988) in the treatment of substance abusing patients.

Although these latter studies do not directly deal with the question of patient-treatment matching, they do serve as a foundation for the formulation of a reasonable and logical assumption that matching one's approach with the individual characteristics and unique problems of the patient might still result in better outcomes.

So, the question remains, "What psychological perspective, along with the therapeutic techniques unique to that perspective, offers the promise of better outcomes in the treatment of substance-reliant individuals?"

The answer is that any psychological perspective, along with the corresponding therapeutic techniques, can be effectively applied to the treatment of addictions so long as it meets the needs of the patient. That's right; nearly all psychotherapeutic techniques work effectively in the treatment of addictions when the techniques applied are matched with the patient's orientation and way of interacting with the environment!

This seems like a rather sweeping statement, does it not? How can such a statement be justified? As sweeping as the statement appears to be, it can be justified by demonstrating that nearly all therapeutic techniques used to treat mental disorders have also been successfully applied to the treatment of addictions. When these techniques have been applied systematically and logically, the results have been positive. This is what prompted researchers to consider the plausibility of patient–treatment matching initially. Let us list some of the therapies applied to substance abuse treatment over the last thirty years.

Earlier in this text, I referred to Hester and Miller's *Handbook of Alcoholism Treatment Approaches: Effective Alternatives, Second Edition* (1995). In this text, the authors, with the assistance of many other researchers, summarily compared the relative effectiveness of thirty-three different substance abuse treatment approaches. Overall, it was demonstrated that brief intervention, social skills training, motivational enhancement, and community reinforcement approaches generally yielded better treatment outcomes than confrontational counseling, psychotherapy, and general alcoholism counseling.

In addition to those techniques recommended by Miller and Hester, rational emotive therapy has been used extensively in the treatment of addictions. Albert Ellis, the originator of this approach, along with other authors, has outlined how this type of therapy is most applicable to the treatment of substance use disorder (Ellis, 1982; Ellis et al., 1988; Ellis and Schoenfield, 1990). Many treatment programs in this country have utilized RET, more recently referred to as rational emotive behavioral therapy (REBT), as a skills-building component to their treatment regimen. Some widely recognized programs such as SMART recovery (Self Management and Recovery Training, 2006–2008) and rational recovery (Jack Trimpey, 2005) have relied heavily on the REBT approach to assist substance-abusing patients. Even the Hazelden Foundation (2008) offers many REBT materials in its bookstore. I have not found any studies that specifically outline how effective REBT is in comparison to other approaches. I believe this is because REBT has frequently been implemented as an adjunct therapy component for other more traditional treatment programs.

Also, REBT is a skills building approach somewhat comparable to the CBST summarized by Hester and Miller (1995).

The applications of the cognitive perspectives are easily found in the treatment of substance use disorders. Aaron Beck et al. (1993) has outlined a thorough and systematic application of cognitive therapy to the treatment of addictions. This approach is described as being a system of psychotherapy which attempts to reduce excessive emotional reactions and self-defeating behavior by modifying faulty thinking and the maladaptive beliefs underlying those reactions.

Another well-known cognitive/behavioral approach to relapse prevention was developed by Marlatt and Gordon (1985). Essentially, the work of these authors proposed that substance-using patients relapse because of their response to high risk stimuli. This approach is designed to correct patients' maladaptive responses.

Although relatively uncommon, psychodynamic approaches to treating substance use disorders have been implemented. In Chapter Seven, Leon Wurmser (1984) proposed that psychoanalytic analysis of the superego was useful to treat the substance-abusing patients' use of mood-altering chemicals in their attempt to avoid feelings and impulses of pain, shame, and anxiety. Edward Khantzian et al. (1990) developed modified dynamic group therapy (MDGT) which was intended to target problems, including affect tolerance, the building of self-esteem, improvement of interpersonal relationships, and the fostering of the development of appropriate self-care strategies. Additionally, Jerome Levin (1987) has outlined a self-psychology approach to treating addictions. This is just to mention a few of the approaches that have come from the psychodynamic perspectives.

Gestalt therapy has been successfully applied to the treatment of addictions (Matzko, 1997; Browne-Miller, 1993). Reality therapy has been much utilized (Glasser, 2000; Carey et al., 1996; Chance et al., 1990). Even dialectical behavioral therapy (Linehan, 1993) has been utilized (Linehan et al., 1999).

I could go on to list more perspectives and approaches. Each of which has proven to be successful when applied to the appropriate patient in the appropriate circumstances.

What does this indicate? It indicates that the treatment of substance use disorders can be approached from any theoretically valid perspective and the attainment of treatment goals can be achieved through the application of a wide range of therapeutic techniques.

Now, this leads us to a much larger and much more important question. If the all these treatment methods have proven to be effective in terms of positive outcomes for patients, why don't we see more treatment programs employ a wider variety of treatment approaches in their efforts to treat substance use disorders?

I can think of two plausible answers.

First, the existing treatment industry is highly invested in, and almost totally dependent upon, the traditional twelve-step approach. It can be said that this traditional approach is all that is available to most people in this nation. Despite the proven ineffectiveness of this treatment method, the addictions treatment industry in this nation continues to rely on the myth that substance dependence is a disease manageable through the application of the mystical twelve-step method.

A second plausible answer is that the overwhelming majority of individuals employed as counselors of substance-abusing patients know little about any treatment method beyond the twelve-step model. In most states, if these counselors are only licensed or certified as chemical dependency counselors, then they are not legally allowed to address any personal issue or problem beyond substance use. These counselors cannot legally offer treatment for problems such as depression, anxiety, personality deficits, or any other psychological factor known to contribute to substance use and abuse.

This brings us to the issue of individualized treatment plans. Do individualized treatment plans exist in the modern treatment of addictions? Actually, they don't exist at all in more than 90 percent of the existing treatment programs. If a treatment program relies on the traditional twelve-step method, there is no need for an individualized treatment plan for any patient. Yes, treatment plans must be created for each individual admitted into treatment. That does not necessarily mean that treatment plans are created specifically to address the unique problems of individual patients.

Twelve-step treatment philosophy assumes that all addicted individuals suffer from a disease—the same disease. According to that philosophy, it's a disease that cannot be cured. It can only be managed. Moreover, it can only be managed if each addicted individual commits to the adherence to the steps and traditions of Alcoholics Anonymous or Narcotics Anonymous. Again, it is a "one tool fixes all" philosophy.

Obviously, when we are talking about treatment plans for a substance use disorder, it is inevitable that we will see that the goals of treatment are similar. For example, in the previous chapter I outlined a set of short-term goals that I believe each patient must attain in order to overcome the reliance upon mood-altering chemicals. There may be some variability regarding goals since not every patient starts treatment from the same place. What makes any treatment plan individualized not only depends upon the specific goals to be attained but also upon the method to be utilized as a means of obtaining those specific goals.

Let us return to the analogy of repairing our beloved BMW. Obviously, any mechanic's treatment goal would likely be to effect a correction of any mechanical malfunction from which our BMW is currently suffering. Let's say that our BMW is found to suffer from a fuel injection problem. It's getting too much gasoline and not enough air in the fuel mixture is getting into the engine's combustion chamber. As such is the case, the engine sputters. Now, fuel injection systems on these vehicles are precise, complex, and delicate. These fuel systems have not only mechanical components but also electrical and computerized controls.

Do we let our "one tool fixes all" mechanic repair our BMW with his five-inch crescent wrench? Probably not! Would it not be a better choice to have a mechanic who has all the tools (a variety of specific wrenches, computerized diagnostic equipment, replacement parts, and so on) needed to repair our vehicle? This latter choice would certainly seem to enhance the chance that our vehicle's problems might be effectively cured. Right?

Again, apply this simple logic to the treatment of an individual patient suffering from a substance use disorder. Any treatment provider's goal is to correct the patient's substance use problem. Just how this patient's substance abuse problem gets resolved depends on all the factors contributing to the development of the patient's problem. All the psychological, social, and environmental influences which have contributed to the development of the substance use problem will need to be dealt with if we are to successfully treat the problem.

Who do you suppose has the best chance of helping this unique substance-disordered individual? Will it likely be the counselor who knows only the traditional twelve-step method of treating substance use problems? Or, will it be the treatment professional that has been adequately trained to approach problems from a variety of valid theoretical perspectives, and can offer treatment which will consist of the application of therapeutic techniques that have established a record of proven efficacy?

Our existing treatment industry still relies on the traditional twelve-step treatment model; there really is no such thing as an individualized treatment plan even though many of these providers make that claim. In most, if not all of these programs, each individual patient must progress to a specified point along the mystical twelve-step path to successfully complete treatment as defined by this approach. It matters not that Joe suffers from severe depression which has contributed to his substance use problems, or that Jan has a history of frequent panic attacks alleviated through the use of copious amounts of alcohol. Joe and Jan both have to complete treatment according to their progress along the twelve-step path. Once Joe and Jan have completed the fourth of the Twelve Steps, as completion of treatment is subjectively defined in most of these programs, their treatment is complete. Essentially, Joe, Jan, or any other patient is prescribed the same treatment regardless of a high variance in contributing factors.

Creating an individualized treatment plan, by comparison, involves a collaborative effort between the primary treatment provider and the patient. This plan not only includes the overall goal of correcting the patient's reliance upon alcohol or other drugs, but it does so in a manner that also addresses the most primary contributors to that substance use problem. It is a plan that is unique for every patient.

Since we are still talking about treating substance use disorders, it makes sense that the primary goal or treatment will be to correct the individuals' reliance upon alcohol and/or other drugs. Short-term treatment goals should still include any or all of those that I had outlined in the previous chapter. But, this is where the similarity between treatment plans for any two specific patients should end.

An individualized treatment plan is like a map. It is an outline, subject to amendment, that not only states overall goal of treatment but also outlines the therapeutic techniques to be utilized. Since each patient comes to treatment with a unique set of problems, life experiences, beliefs, opinions, outlook, and world view, this plan will vary from one patient to another.

To illustrate what an individualized treatment plan might look like, let us take a look at a plan intended to assist a single patient (Joe) to attain the first short-term goal of substance abuse treatment:

Primary Goal of Treatment
Eliminate Joe's psychological reliance upon alcohol.

Short-Term Goal That Leads to Primary Goal
Constructively address Joe's denial of the problems that have contributed to his use of alcohol. Joe admits that he has a problem with alcohol. Joe does not verbally acknowledge that he uses alcohol as a means to alleviate symptoms of depression.

Intervention
Application of reality therapy techniques will be employed in an effort to demonstrate that a real connection exists between Joe's use of alcohol and his effort to avoid feelings of helplessness and hopelessness.

Behavioral Objectives of Intervention
Joe will journalize the last five occasions that he used alcohol to excess complete with a description of what he was thinking and feeling just prior to, during, and after his use of alcohol. Joe will, in brief written form, illustrate the connection that exists between what he was thinking and feeling and his use of alcohol on each of these five occasions. Additionally, Joe will verbalize his responsibility for engaging in the use of alcohol. This will be discussed with his primary therapist in individual counseling, and it will be presented in group therapy. Joe

will verbally acknowledge in individual and group therapy that he uses alcohol as one means of alleviating his depression, and that he alone is responsible for that behavior.

As can be seen, this is a simple plan to achieve one short-term goal. It does, however, provide a complete description of what is to be accomplished and how the patient will accomplish specific objectives that will lead him to the attainment of a specific short-term goal. This is a plan that specifically addresses the needs of this individual patient.

A treatment plan created for Jan, who suffered panic attacks, would certainly include the same overall goal and probably the same short term goal if Jan still suffers from denial. But, the similarity between Joe and Jan's plan would end there. Jan suffers from panic attacks, not depression. Jan's problem might be more effectively dealt with by approaching her problems from a different theoretical perspective. Therefore, different therapeutic techniques would be employed to assist Jan to achieve a set of objectives more relevant to her problems.

An example of an appropriate treatment plan for Jan might be as follows:

Primary Goal of Treatment
Eliminate Jan's psychological reliance upon alcohol.

Short-Term Goal That Leads to Primary Goal
Jan has acknowledged that she uses mood-altering chemicals as a means of alleviating symptoms she describes as being panic attacks. Jan has not been able to verbally describe why certain events or circumstances trigger these attacks. The short-term goal will be to assist Jan to make the cognitive connections that lay between the events and circumstances which trigger feelings of anxiety and thereby cause Jan to experience an urge to use mood-altering chemicals.

Intervention
Application of cognitive therapy techniques will be utilized to assist Jan to identify her core beliefs that, when stimulated, cause Jan to experience feelings of anxiety and trigger her urge to use mood-altering chemicals.

Behavioral Objectives of Intervention
Jan will be able to diagram the core beliefs she maintains, the automatic thoughts that occur to her when she is exposed to specific events or circumstances, the emotions she experiences in those instances, and addictive beliefs and conclusions that lead to her desire to use mood-altering chemicals. Jan will seek assistance in creating her diagram in group therapy, and she will discuss her diagrams with her primary therapist.

According to what is outlined in this, Jan's current treatment plan, it is obvious that Jan has dealt with the issue of denial. The current short-term goal in Jan's treatment is essentially to assist Jan to make the connection between her use of mood-altering substances and her desire to escape troublesome thoughts and emotions (STG #2, as outlined in Chapter Thirteen). This, according to the primary therapist's clinical judgment, can best be accomplished through the application of therapeutic techniques taken from the cognitive perspective. Jan can behaviorally demonstrate that she is attaining this short term goal by accurately diagramming what she believes about herself, what she experiences when she is exposed to distressing events and circumstances, and why all this triggers her desire to use drugs and/or alcohol.

Treatment plans should always provide this type of a map for both the patient and the treatment service providers. Specific individualized treatment plans are needed to keep the patient and the treatment service providers focused upon what a patient needs to accomplish, how this is to be accomplished, and what needs to be observed of a patient as a demonstration that objectives have been completed and specific goals have been attained.

As previously stated, treatment providers need to have many tools. There is no one tool that fixes the all the problems contributing to the development of substance use disorders in all individuals. Therapists and other professionals who provide services in the addictions treatment field need to be fully educated and adequately trained to be able to approach any individual patient's problems from a variety of theoretically valid perspectives. Treatment professionals then have to be able to employ therapeutic techniques that will effectively meet the needs of the individual patient. Above all, this needs to be done in a logical and systematic manner.

So, we are back to our original question. What approach and set of therapeutic techniques work best in the treatment of addictions?

The answer is: they all work in the right place, at the right time, with the right patient. Yes, gestalt therapy, client-centered therapy, reality therapy, psychodynamic therapies, cognitive therapies, behavioral therapies, and so on can all be utilized effectively in the treatment of substance use disorders. Furthermore, applications of these various forms of therapy frequently prove to be much more effective than traditional twelve-step treatment.

All theoretically valid perspectives along with the therapeutic techniques derived from these perspectives have something to offer in the treatment of substance use disorders. There are some important qualifications that must be placed on this statement. How well any therapeutic technique works depends on the following qualifying factors: 1. how well the technique directly addresses the psychological problems exhibited by the individual patient; 2. whether the technique matches the individual patient's characteristic style of relating to the world; and 3. how skilled is the therapist or counselor in the provision of the technique to be applied.

References

Chapter Fourteen

Beck, A. A., Wright, F. D., Newman, C. F., and Liese, B. S. (1993). *Cognitive Therapy of Substance Abuse.* New York, NY: Guilford Press.

Beck, A. T., Steer, R. A., and Brown, G. K. (1996). *Manual for the Beck Depression Inventory-II.* San Antonio, TX: Psychological Corporation.

Browne-Miller, A. (1993). *Gestalting Addiction: The Addiction-focused Group Therapy of Dr. Richard Louis Miller.* Norwood, NJ: Ablex Publishing Corporation.

Bufe, C. (1998). How Effective is AA? *Alcoholics Anonymous: Cult or Cure.* 2nd edition, revised. San Francisco, CA: See Sharp Press.

Canton, G., Giannini, L., Magni, G., Bertinaria, A., Cibin, M., and Gallimerti, L. (1988). Locus of control, life events and treatment outcome in alcohol dependent patients. *Acta Psychiatrica Scandinavica,* **78**, 18–23.

Carey, T. A., Farrell-Jones, M., and Rowan, H. S. (1996). What do you really want? A control theory/reality therapy approach to understanding alcoholism. *Journal of Reality Therapy,* **16(1)**, 3–18.

Chance, E., Bibens, R. F., Cowley, J., Pouretedal, M., Dolese, P., and Virtue, D. (1990). A drug/alcohol treatment program for negatively addicted inmates. *Journal of Reality Therapy,* **9(2),** 33–38.

Cloninger, C. R. (1987). *The Tridimensional Personality Questionnaire, Version IV.* St. Louis, MO: Washington University School of Medicine.

Ellis, A. (1982). The treatment of alcohol and drug abuse: A rational emotive approach. *Rational Living,* **17(2)**, 15–24.

Ellis, A., and Schoenfeld, E. (1990). Divine intervention and the treatment of chemical dependency. *Journal of Substance Abuse,* **2**, 459–468.

Ellis, A., McInerey, J. F., DiGuiseppe, R., and Yeager, R. J. (1988). *Rational Emotive Therapy with Alcoholics and Substance Abusers.* New York, NY: Pergamon Press.

Ewing, J. (1984). Detecting alcoholism: The CAGE questionnaire. *JAMA,* **252(14)**, 905–1907.

Franzke, L. H., Clifford, P. A., and Maisto, S. A. (2001). Alcohol treatment outcomes and social functioning: Testing a matching hypothesis. Paper presented at the 129th meeting of the American Public Health Association. Department of Health Studies, New York University.

Glasser, W. (2000). *Reality therapy in action.* New York, NY: Harper Collins Publishers.

Gordis, E. (1997). Patient-treatment matching. A commentary by NIAAA Director, Enoch Gordis, MD. *Alcohol Alert,* No. 36.

Hamilton, M. (1960) A rating scale for depression. *Journal of Neurology, Neurosurgery, and Psychiatry,* **23**, 56–62.

Hazelden Foundation, 2008. Hazelden bookstore. Web site: http://www.hazalden.org.

Khantzian, E. J., Halliday, K. S., and McAuliffe, W. E. (1990). *Addiction and the Vulnerable Self: Modified Dynamic Group Therapy for Substance Abusers.* New York, NY: Guilford Press.

Levin, J. D. (1987). *Treatment of Alcoholism and Other Addictions: A Self-Psychology Approach.* Northvale, NJ: Jason Aronson Inc.

Linehan, M. M. (1993). *Cognitive Behavioral Treatment of Borderline Personality Disorder.* New York, NY: Guilford Press.

Linehan, M. M., Schmidt, H., Dimeff, L. A., Kanter, J. W., Craft, J. C., Comtois, K. A., and Recknor, K. L. (1999). Dialectical behavior therapy for patients with borderline personality disorder and drug-dependence. *American Journal on Addiction,* **8**, 279–292.

Marlatt, G. A., and Gordon, J. R. (1985). *Relapse Prevention: Maintenance Strategies in the Treatment of Addictive Behaviors.* New York, NY: Guilford Press.

Mattson, M. E. (1994). Patient-treatment matching. *Alcohol Health and Research World,* **18(4)**, 287–295.

Matzko, H. (1997). A gestalt therapy treatment approach for addictions: Multi-phasic transformational process. (pp. 34–55) *Gestalt Review* 1/1.

Miller, W. R., and Rollnick, S. (2002). *Motivational Interviewing: Preparing people for change. 2nd Ed.* New York, NY: Guilford Press.

Meyers, I., and McCaulley, M. (1985). *A Guide to the Development and Use of the Meyers-Briggs Type Indicator.* Palo Alto, CA: Consulting Psychologists Press.

Myers, I. B., McCaulley, M. H., Quenk, N. L., and Hammer, A. L. (1998). *MBTI Manual (A guide to the development and use of the*

Myers Briggs type indicator). 3rd ed. Consulting Psychologists Press.

Peele, S. (1998). Ten radical things NIAAA research shows about alcoholism. *The Addictions Newsletter.* (pp. 6, 17-19) The American Psychological Association, Division 50. Spring 1998. Vol. 5, No.2.

Project MATCH Research Group. (1993). Project Match: Rationale and methods for a multisite clinical trial matching patients to alcoholism treatment. *Alcoholism: Clinical and Experimental Research,* **17**, 1130–1145.

Project MATCH Research Group. (1997). Matching alcoholism treatments to client heterogeneity: Project Match Posttreatment drinking outcomes. *Journal of Studies on Alcohol,* **58**, 7–29.

Roman, P., and Blum, T. (1997). National Treatment Summary Report. (p. 20) Athens, GA: Institute for Behavioral Research.

Self Management and Recovery Training, 2006–2008. Web site: http://www.smartrecovery.org.

Sellman, J. D., Mulder, R. T., Sullivan, P. F., and Joyce, P. R. (1997). Low persistence predicts relapse in alcohol dependence following treatment. *Journal of Studies on Alcohol,* **58**, 257–263.

Selzer, M. L. (1971). The Michigan Alcoholism Screening Test (MAST): The Quest for a New Diagnostic Instrument. *American Journal of Psychiatry,* **127**, 1653–1658.

Spielberger, C. D., and Gorsuch, R. L. (1983). *Manual for the State-trait anxiety inventory (form Y) ("self-evaluation questionnaire").* Palo Alto, CA: Consulting Psychologists Press.

Tarnai, J., and Young, F. L. (1983). Alcoholic's personalities: extrovert or introvert? *Psychological Reports,* **53**, 123–127.

Timko, C., and Sempel, J. M. (2004). Short-term outcomes of matching dual diagnosis patients' symptom severity to treatment intensity. *Journal of Substance Abuse Treatment,* **26**, 209–218.

Trimpey, J. (2005). Rational Recovery. Website: http://www.rational.org.

Willinger,U., Lenzinger, E., Hornik, K., Fischer, G., Schonbeck, G, Aschauer, H. N., and Meszaros, K. (2002). Anxiety as a predictor of relapse in detoxified alcohol dependent patients. *Alcohol and Alcoholism,* **37(6)**, 609–612.

Wurmser, L. (1984). The role of superego conflicts in substance abuse and their treatment. *International Journal of Psychoanalytic Psychotherapy,* **10**, 227–258.

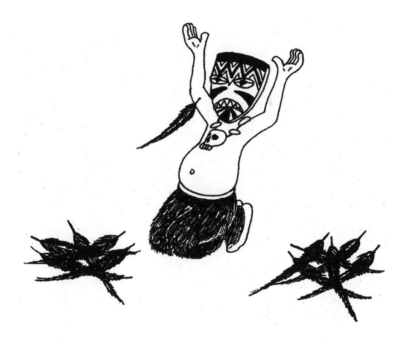

Chapter 15

Relapse and Relapse Prevention

No discussion of the treatment of substance use disorders would be complete without addressing the issue of relapse. Anyone in the treatment field knows that patient relapse is a problem to be addressed with regard to all patients. The most predictable outcome of traditional treatment of addictions is relapse. Estimates of patient relapse vary greatly. Commonly, it is estimated that for both outpatient and residential treatment programs approximately 50 percent of patients relapse within one to two months of beginning treatment (Hunt et al., 1971; O'Malley et al., 1992; Volpicelli et al., 1992).

Now, this is pretty dismal in terms of outcome. We have discussed various estimates as to outcome of treatment in previous chapters of this text. I will not rehash these numbers. Suffice it to say that the existing empirical evidence indicates that current and past treatments for substance use disorders have been ineffective. Even no treatment at all is at least as effective as traditional treatment!

Let's compare a 50 percent relapse rate in relation to any other illness. Would it be an acceptable outcome if 50 percent of all patients undergoing angioplasty procedures to prevent death from heart disease collapsed from heart attacks within two months of experiencing this procedure? Not likely. Would be acceptable if more than 50 percent of individuals who threaten suicide actually commit suicide within two months of getting intervention? Certainly not! How about treatment for depression? Anxiety? Or any illness?

If going through any form of treatment for any illness, disorder, or malady was equivalent to a coin toss in terms of outcome, why bother? There's a fifty-fifty chance you get better with no treatment at all. Essentially, this is what we see regarding the existing treatment industry in this nation. Then, when you add that only a very small percentage of individuals who actually suffer from substance use disorders ever even seek formal treatment, and that approximately nine out of ten individuals who attend twelve-step groups in an effort to overcome their problems drop out within a period of a few months, outcomes become even more questionable.

So what does this mean in terms of relapse and relapse prevention? It means that the individuals who repeatedly relapse shortly after having undergone treatment never actually received treatment for their substance use problems in the first place. If their problems had been definitively treated, these individuals would not be constantly relapsing.

No individual who seeks treatment for a substance use disorder should ever be said to have successfully completed treatment if the treatment provider has reason to believe that the individual will likely relapse as soon as he or she exits the treatment facility.

The exact point of treatment is to eliminate the substance-abusing behavior and replace it with behavior that is more functional and constructive. If this isn't being accomplished, no treatment has occurred.

References

Chapter Fifteen

Hunt, W. A., Barnett, L. W. and Brach, L. G. (1971). Relapse rates in addiction programs. *Journal of Clinical Psychology,* **27**, 455–456.

O'Malley, S. S., Jaffe, A. J., Chang, G., Schottenfeld, R. S., Meyer, R. E., and Rounsaville, B. (1992). Naltrexone and coping skills therapy for alcohol dependence. *Archives of General Psychiatry,* **49**, 881–887.

Volpicelli, J. R., Alterman, A. I., Hayashida, M., and O'Brien, C. P. (1992). Naltrexone in the treatment of alcohol dependence. *Archives of General Psychiatry,* **49**, 876–880.

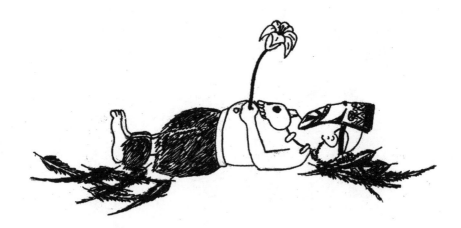

Manufactured By: RR Donnelley
                     Momence, IL USA
                     August , 2010